Formulation in Mental H

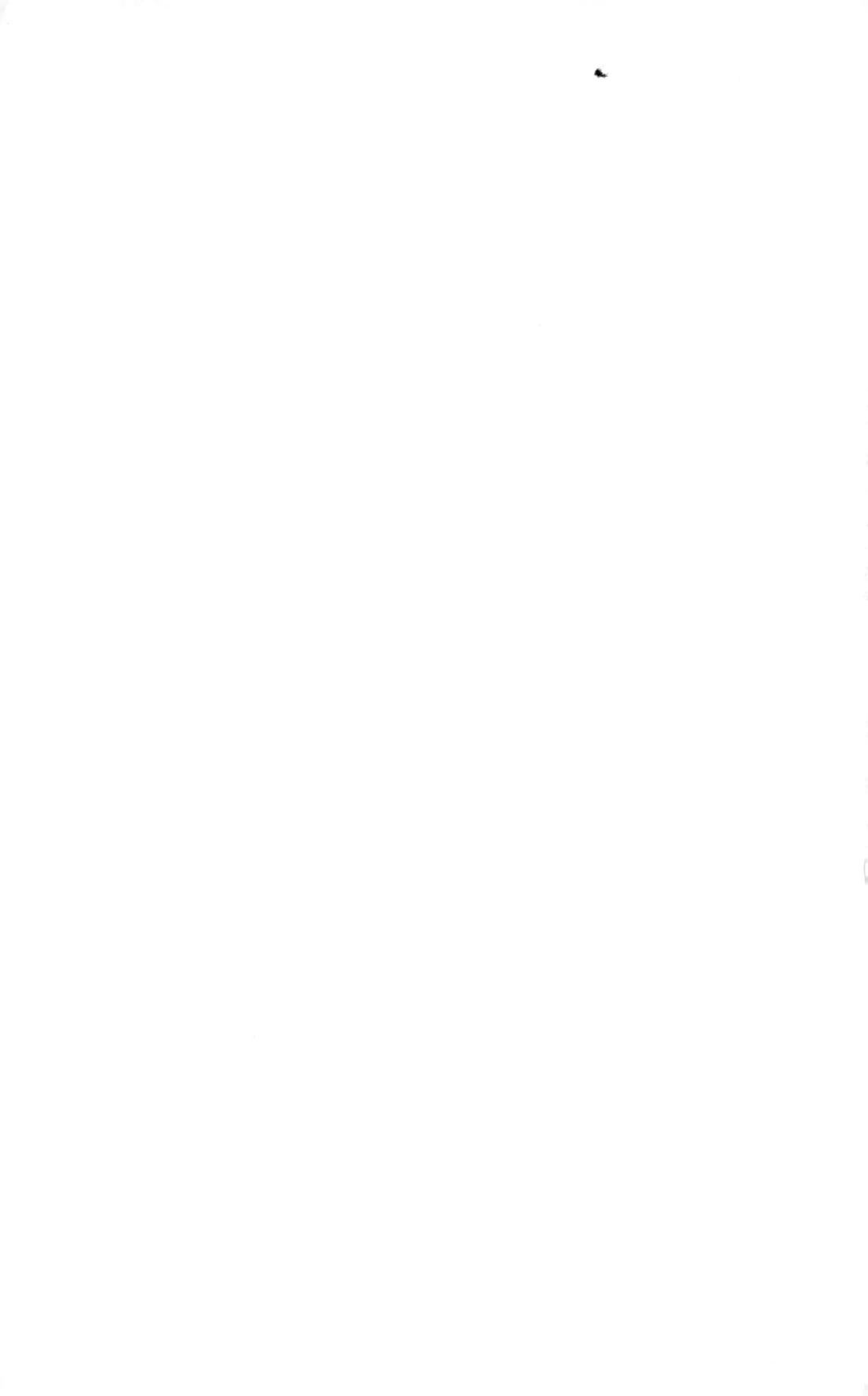

Vickie Howard • Lolita Alfred
Editors

Formulation in Mental Health Nursing

palgrave
macmillan

Editors
Vickie Howard
Faculty of Health Sciences
University of Hull
Hull, UK

Lolita Alfred
School of Health and Psychological
Sciences
City, University of London
London, UK

ISBN 978-3-031-59955-2   ISBN 978-3-031-59956-9   (eBook)
https://doi.org/10.1007/978-3-031-59956-9

Cover illustration: LEOcrafts/Getty Images

This Palgrave Macmillan imprint is published by the registered company Springer Nature
Switzerland AG.
The registered company address is: Gewerbestrasse 11, 6330 Cham, Switzerland

If disposing of this product, please recycle the paper.

ACKNOWLEDGEMENTS

We would like to thank academic and clinical practice colleagues for the valuable conversations and insights that stimulated our thinking and shaped how we have written this book. We would also like to thank the students who have contributed to identifying the gaps that this book has consequently sought to fill. This has involved exploring how we can enhance the role that mental health nursing and mental health nurses as members of the multidisciplinary team can play to support person centred, and family centred recovery through formulation.

We would also like to thank all the individuals we have worked with over the years for inspiring us, deepening our learning and desire for working in a hope-filled way, and enhancing our compassion for people who are experiencing emotional distress.

We are grateful to our Commissioning Editor Clelia Petracca and our Book Editorial Manager Bhavya Rattan for their ongoing support, guidance and help to get us across that finish line! We would also like to thank the peer-reviewers for their time, expertise, ideas, and all-round invaluable feedback which helped to enhance our work at the book proposal stage and at the final manuscript stage.

To our chapter authors and contributors—we thank you for sharing this journey with us—for all your time, thoughts and contributions. It would not have been possible to produce this book without your valuable contributions.

And finally, to our families and friends—we thank you for keeping us grounded and bearing with us while we took moments of time away from you to focus on this book.

CONTENTS

Notes on Contributors

Amina Adan is a lecturer and researcher at the Tavistock and Portman NHS Trust. Dr Adan has an interest in the application of psychodynamic and psychosocial thinking and practice in the public sphere. More broadly, her research interests include the exploration of contemporary perspectives on the complex issue of gendered violence.

Lolita Alfred is a senior lecturer at City, University of London, and a senior fellow of the Higher Education Academy. She has been registered as a mental health nurse for 20 years and she has clinical experience as a facilitator of substance use/substance-related offending therapy and using Cognitive Behaviour Therapy-based approaches. She has led (and taught) undergraduate and postgraduate modules on Cognitive Behaviour Therapy and Formulation. She is passionate about supporting learners to develop knowledge and understanding of emotional and psychological distress, the various theories that might explain different experiences, and the role and relevance of formulation to support compassionate care and person-centred recovery. Dr Alfred has a PhD in Public Health and is a member of the Editorial Board for the International Journal of Drug Policy, and she peer-reviews papers for several journals on mental health and substance use. Her research interests and publications to date centre around alcohol use across the lifespan, mental health and public health.

Claire Barber is a senior lecturer in Mental Health at City, University of London, and a fellow of the Higher Education Academy. She is a postgraduate programme director and leads and teaches continuing professional development (CPD) standalone Master's level modules on child and adolescent mental health and liaison mental health care. She also teaches on the preregistration BSc and MSc programmes in the Nursing Division. She has been registered as a mental health nurse for nearly 30 years. She is a systemic psychotherapist, trained at the Tavistock and Portman NHS Foundation Trust, London. Claire also works privately providing therapy for children, young people, families, couples, individual adults, groups and adoption / fostering families who are experiencing emotional difficulties, trauma survivors, mental health diagnosis and relationship difficulties. She is also involved in organisational consultancy and training. She regularly facilitates group clinical supervision for health and social care professionals across a variety of teams and organisations. Claire is a member of the Association of Family Therapists and a full clinical member of the United Kingdom Council for Psychotherapy.

Michelle Gideon is an NMC registered mental health nurse, obtaining her BSc from London Southbank University and has been in practice for nearly 20 years. She has worked in a number of different NHS settings such as: Mental Health Liaison within A&E, Early Intervention Services, the Home Treatment Team, the Crisis Therapy Service and many years as a care co-ordinator for recovery teams across London. Currently, she works as a first contact mental health practitioner, a dual role sitting between primary and secondary mental healthcare services. In 2022, Michelle completed her MSc in Psychology at the University of East London with her dissertation focusing on the lived experiences of black, bisexual women in London. More recently, she finished additional MSc modules in Psychopharmacology at Middlesex University and Physical Health Needs in Mental Health at London Southbank University. Her final project focused on co-morbidities of obesity within patients with Schizophrenia and offered some considerations for future practice. Michelle is a clinical supervisor and provides training to 3rd year Advanced Diploma Counselling students in the areas of psychiatry, psychopathology and psychodynamics.

Claire Grainger has over 20 years' experience of working in the NHS and as a registered mental health nurse. During this time, Claire went on to undertake a further degree in Specialist Community Public Health Nursing which allowed her to become dual trained as a health visitor. Claire has experience of working in Child and Adolescent Mental Health Services, currently Named Nurse for Children in Care and Team Leader for the Children in Care Team at Rotherham, Doncaster and South Humber NHS Trust.

Georgia Grainger has recently graduated from university, achieving a first-class honours in Early Childhood Studies. She is now pursuing her PGCE in Early Childhood Education and Care (0–5) with early years' teacher status to gain employment as a primary school teacher. She is a true inspiration to everyone around her.

Vickie Howard is a lecturer and deputy programme director for the Mental Health and Wellbeing Practitioner Programme at the University of Hull. She registered as a mental health nurse in 1997 and has worked in a number of clinical, leadership and managerial posts. Her interests in psychologically informed interventions started with the completion of The Thorn Diploma in Problem Centred Interventions and she has since studied in the areas of psychotherapy, counselling and hypnotherapy. In 2016, she moved to an academic post as a lecturer in mental health nursing at the University of Hull, progressing to the role of Programme Director for BSc Mental Health Nursing

Apprenticeships. She is currently working towards a PhD by Published Works and studying for an MSc in Psychology. Her research interests involve the therapeutic use of self, clinical supervision and narcissistic abuse/pathological relationships. Vickie is also a counsellor and clinical supervisor in private practice and was awarded the Queen's Nurse title in 2023.

Naomi Marlow is a creative person with a love for arts and crafts. She likes finding spaces to enjoy and has a few bases where she spends her time. She appreciates nature and takes joy in it.

Michelle Martin is a registered mental health nurse and lecturer at the University of Hull. Michelle has experience of clinical practice within acute adult inpatient settings and community mental health services. She has an interest in co-occurring mental health and substance use and holds experience of clinical work within the area of dual diagnosis. Michelle also has an interest in health and social care leadership, specifically the experiences of staff and the impact these have on mental healthcare delivery. Michelle completed her Master's in Health and Social Care Leadership at the York St John University in 2023.

Roselyne Masamha is a staff development consultant with a doctorate in clinical education. She is a senior fellow of the Advanced Higher Education (SFHEA) and currently an honorary research fellow at the University of Exeter. She has held a variety of nursing roles, including that of Clinical Nurse Specialist in forensic learning disability secure settings, where she supported individuals with a dual diagnosis of learning disabilities and mental ill-health, at the interface of the Criminal Justice System and Mental Health Law. The individuals she supported as part of a wider multidisciplinary team had highly complex presentations which required collaborative working and interprofessional input to ensure rounded and effective care interventions. Dr Roselyne Masamha is also an independent researcher—whose expertise is grounded in the concepts of knowledge production, specifically the insights that marginalised knowledges bring to mainstream, dominant understandings. Her published works span across mental health, clinical supervision, migration, knowledge production and decolonial tensions.

Charity Mudimu is a registered mental health nurse currently working as Lead Nurse for Health and Wellbeing on a joint post across East London NHS Foundation Trust and City, University of London. This role has seen her promote wellbeing, help colleagues and students to successfully achieve their academic and clinical practice goals. Charity has over 20 years' experience working in various settings and using a range of psychologically informed approaches including Open Dialogue. She is particularly passionate about working in Acute Community Crisis Resolution Home Treatment Teams and Crisis Lines, and has held various nursing and leadership roles, including more recently, as manager of a Crisis Resolution team. Charity is passionate about helping clients to manage any crisis they might be in, empowering and supporting them to reach their full potential.

Jane Peirson is a senior lecturer in Mental Health Nursing at York St John University, teaching undergraduate nursing. She has an MSc in Community Nursing and is a Queen's Nurse. She has over 20 years' experience as a registered mental health nurse working in various mental health settings. After recognising a trend in the theme of childhood trauma impacting on a person's mental health outcomes, she retrained as a specialist community public health nurse—health visitor to provide earlier intervention in supporting young families and children. She has an interest in areas of perinatal and infant mental health, mental health trauma and the longer-term impacts on the person's health and wellbeing outcomes.

Betty Williamson has lived alongside severe mental illness for several years and now actively uses her lived experience as a mental health service user to facilitate teaching on self-harm and suicide, working with staff from various organisations including schools. She also lectures at a university for several of their health and social care degree programmes. Betty has an extensive background which includes work with The Royal College of Psychiatrists (RCOP) project 'Better Services for People who Self Harm', providing a service user perspective for both local services and other hospitals. She has also worked with the RCOP as a service user consultant for PLAN (Psychiatric Liaison Accreditation Network). She has served as a non-executive director at a mental health trust and worked with Skills for Care and Health on the Positive and Safe Initiative. Betty has a body of published work on her lived experience and has been a guest keynote speaker at several conferences including: Restraint Reduction Network: Examining What Works, the Design in Mental Health Conference, Positive and Safe Conference, Department of Health and Royal College of Nursing Conferences. She is a passionate believer in co-production and has published on the subject.

ABBREVIATIONS

ACEs   Adverse Childhood Experiences
AMHP   Approved Mental Health Practitioner
APIE   Assessment, Planning, Implementation, Evaluation
APTI   Anti-Pathologising Trauma Informed Services
BPPS   Biopsychopharmasocial
BPS   British Psychological Society
BtC   Behaviours that Challenge
CAT   Cognitive Analytic Therapy
CBT   Cognitive Behavioural Therapy
CHIME   Connectedness, Hope, Identity, Meaning, Empowerment
CMHN   Community Mental Health Nurse
CPD   Continuing Professional Development
DBT   Dialectical Behavioural Therapy
DSM   Diagnostic Statistical Manual
EI   Early Intervention
EIP   Early Intervention in Psychosis
HEE   Health Education England
IAPT   Improving Access to Psychological Therapies
ICB   Integrated Care Board
ICD   International Classification of Diseases
ITIM   Indicative Trauma Impact Manual
MHN   Mental Health Nurse
MHWP   Mental Health and Wellbeing Practitioner
NHS   National Health Service
NICE   National Institute for Health and Care Excellence
NMC   Nursing and Midwifery Council
NMHT   Neighbourhood Mental Health Team
NPD   Narcissistic Personality Disorder
PSI   Psychosocial Interventions
PTMF   Power Threat Meaning Framework
PWP   Psychological Wellbeing Practitioner
TIC   Trauma Informed Care

LIST OF FIGURES

LIST OF TABLES

Understanding Human Distress and an Invitation to Explore the Myriads of Formulation

Vickie Howard and Lolita Alfred

Key Learning Points
- An introduction to the book and its layout
- Exploring the use of language and terminology
- Outlining the multitude of ways to understand human emotional and psychological distress with reference to historical and current developments
- Underpinning theory and approaches to formulation
- An exploration of the contributions that mental health nursing can make

Welcome to Chap. 1 which focuses on introducing the key sources of underpinning concepts in developing formulation approaches in mental health nursing. These will be further explored and illustrated through the real-life accounts within subsequent chapters of this book. We are aiming to present these concepts in straightforward and accessible language to support you with your own sense-making and applications of these theories and concepts, and we begin

V. Howard
Faculty of Health Sciences, University of Hull, Hull, UK
e-mail: V.Howard@Hull.ac.uk

L. Alfred (✉)
City, University of London, London, UK
e-mail: Lolita.Alfred@city.ac.uk

V. Howard, L. Alfred (eds.), *Formulation in Mental Health Nursing*,
https://doi.org/10.1007/978-3-031-59956-9_1

below by outlining our intentions with language use for the writing style and presentation of the book. Ultimately, we hope this introductory information will spark your individual areas of interest and that you will begin the journey of 'making (mental) notes' on the specific approaches and viewpoints you may naturally align to and recognise others which may be unfamiliar yet possibly intriguing! This first chapter will provide the highlights of historical developments and current thinking in how human distress has been viewed and named, and consequently the reactions to how distress should be addressed and intervened with.

Key influencing theoretical literature and research will be reflected upon in relation to what may support and help the distressed individual. Ultimately, the question will be asked regarding what considerations does all this lead to for mental health nursing practice and specifically inquire if we can begin piecing together the characteristics of what formulation in mental health nursing and by mental health nurses in differing roles looks like. We are proposing a definition at the outset of this book that formulation in mental health nursing practice is '*a collaborative and therapeutic process between person and helper which supports an exploration of sources of distress and discussions of what to do about it*'.

A Note on Language, Terminology and How This Book Is Written

What becomes apparent when writing about distress is that there are many phrases and words which can be and are used to describe this psychological state. Throughout this text, words such as 'mental health problems', 'mental distress', and 'mental illness', will be used to describe the distressed state. The choice of these words will depend on the perspective of distress we are writing from and a person's choice of language, for example although mental illness is often used in conjunction with the medical and psychiatric model and in relation to diagnostic criteria, it may also be the choice of someone with a lived experience of mental distress to use this term.

At the very beginning, when we were putting forward our ideas and plans for this book and produced a formal book proposal for the publisher, one of the anonymous reviewers highlighted that although our goal was to incorporate a more trauma informed perspective to the ethos of our book, we still referred to or slipped back into a medical model language without rationale on occasion. We appreciated this feedback as it prompted us to reflect on the underlying complexities of why we did this. We deduce that as mental health nurses, both of us (Vickie and Lolita) have worked in heavily underpinned medical model mental healthcare environments, (as well as more user-led and nurse-led ones which arguably incorporated more recovery-focused language—more on recovery-focused language later). We therefore recognise we have an eclectic amalgamation of the language we use, and we have integrated our nursing practice within the medical/psychiatric model because that was the overriding approach of a good portion of the services we have worked within. It was also 'the norm' as a therapeutic process for the assessment and treatment of what were/are commonly referred to as mental health problems. It is likely that this may be the experience of many of our readers and we do not want to marginalise our readers by saying terms like 'mental illness', 'mentally unwell' should not be used, when these are the predominant terms used within many areas of current practice, care environments and wider society. We also appreciate that different cultural and environmental perspectives can influence terminology used and with this in mind, there will be a mix of terminology used in this book (depending on author style) however we do not purport to use all terminology possible within this book. What we feel is more important, is for the individual, nurse/practitioner or student reading this book to reflect on their own use of language and that of the service and context they work within and to have these discussions with colleagues, to work towards any changes in outlooks and language use which may appear indicated. Although language is an important consideration (shaping attitudes and therapeutic approaches)—what may be more important to the distressed person is feeling respected, listened to, and genuinely cared for rather than us getting tied up about whether we are expressing the currently considered 'correct term'. In addition, some people experiencing distress may relate to and prefer medical/psychiatric language because it defines, describes, and validates their experiences in a manner which makes sense to them and their families and friends. We also want to provide a bit of an explanation regarding how we have approached the writing of this book and how we value the diversity of the contributing chapter authors. We very much want to be 'in conversation' with you as readers, when possible, to spark your views and ideas on the issues raised. You will see that the chapter authors will have their own styles and ways of presenting their discussions, but with a consistent aim of including 'the person's experiences of distress' as the essential thread in linking discussions and making their experiences the central focus. To facilitate this, throughout, we employ a narrative inquiry style, whereby we are placing the person's autobiographical experiences as key areas for exploration. We also draw on the chapter authors' and contributors' experiences—whether this is from an academic, practitioner or service user/lived experience perspective. In addition, we borrow from autoethnography which has been described as '...*an autobiographical genre of writing and research that displays multiple layers of consciousness, connecting the personal to the cultural*' (Bochner & Ellis, 2016, p. 65). In many instances throughout this book, we are bearing witness to an individual's experiences and applying compassion in our approaches, again taking inspiration from Carolyn Ellis's autoethnographic research which resulted in a connection with others as well as an aim towards the realisation of social justice (Ellis, 2017). By fully involving an individual (and in some instances, family members/carers/friends) who is sharing their autobiographical experiences within the chapters, we collaborate in the formulation being developed. In addition, as a priority we want to hear people's views, reflections and individual experiences relating to the wider cultural, societal and possibly political backgrounds which may have shaped and influenced their experiences and interpretations. This fits well with current outlooks in both mental health nursing education and practice which view co-production (involving nurses, service users and their families) as an essential component of developing and retaining the mental health nursing workforce (NHS Health Education England, 2022). So, let's begin by looking at some interpretations of human distress:

THE FORMULATION OF HUMAN DISTRESS AND HOW PHILOSOPHY, ONTOLOGY AND EPISTEMOLOGY HAVE INFLUENCED MENTAL HEALTH NURSING PERSPECTIVES

This section could be a book in its own right and as there are many books which have focused on the history of distress; we refer to a few examples here as 'the history of madness and mental health' (Eghigian, 2019), 'women and madness' (Chessler, 2018) and 'a history of psychiatry: from the era of the asylum to the age of prozac' (Shorter, 1997). Included are fascinating accounts and propositions of how those suffering and displaying unusual behaviours were viewed throughout history by the majority of society and how they were treated. Reading a selection of these texts automatically brings the obvious and most burning question many of us strive to know the answer to … are the approaches and outlooks towards those suffering distress (and showing unusual behaviours) much better, more humane and less damaging in the society we live in today? We would surely think that they must be with ongoing scientific progression and the ethos of 'evidence-based practice' where interventions are proposed to be based on the use of current best evidence in combination with clinical expertise and patient values (Jennings & Loan, 2001; Titler, 2006). However, this section will take us through a whistle stop exploration, pausing for some critical enquiry along the way where maybe surface suppositions may not be so clear cut about contemporary mental health care. We will then discuss these historical considerations in relation to mental health nursing and its course and development. Those texts exploring and presenting historical outlooks on mental distress clearly present the changes in language and accepted viewpoints which have been used to describe the distressed individual. These relate to epistemological, ontological and overarching philosophical underpinnings at particular points in time.

The field of mental health care is one of competing paradigms and understandings about what constitutes mental health and mental illness (Crowe et al., 2008). The very nature and validity of mental health conditions and applied diagnosis is an example of an area that is viewed from different perspectives (we expand on this in the section on developments in mental health within this chapter). To begin exploring how we have come to have these different paradigms and understandings in mental health—we must first understand *Epistemology*—which is defined as a branch of philosophy that is concerned with '*the theory of knowledge*' (Crotty, 1998, p. 3). In other words, epistemology is a way of understanding and explaining how we know the things that we know. It prompts consideration of why we believe or hold certain views, and how we justify the positions we take on a particular topic or area. Applying this to the example of mental health or mental illness, one epistemological question we might ask is '*How do we know what we know about mental health or mental illness?*' And to answer this, we might gather 'knowledge' about what mental health and mental illness is without experience (also known as '*a priori*' knowledge). We can, however, also have knowledge gained through our experience of events or circumstances (also known as '*a posteriori*' knowledge). It is also worth mentioning that knowledge or what we know can change over time (we explore mental health history and change over time later in this chapter). Furthermore, what we know can also be influenced by place/environment, culture and social norms amongst other factors. For example, what is viewed as 'hearing voices' or 'psychosis' in one culture, may be viewed by another culture as an expression of spirituality, and in another culture, it may be understood as 'witchcraft' or 'possession'.

The other concept to consider as part of unpacking how we have come to have different understandings of mental health and mental illness is the concept of '*Ontology*'. Ontology is defined as the study of objects and their relationships. It is concerned with the nature and structure of '*reality*', or '*what is*' (Crotty, 1998, p. 10). To make the definition of ontology less abstract, Brabazon (2023) offers an analogy of ontology as the concrete foundation of a house—to have a house that is sturdy, it must have a solid foundation on which it is built. Once the building of the house is complete, most people will see the house, but not necessarily the concrete foundations beneath it. With this in mind, for us to understand what mental health is (the house analogy), our understanding of it must be built on a solid foundation, with due consideration of the parts that make up the foundation, and the relationship of the parts within the foundation. Ontology as a branch of philosophy acknowledges there can be a dichotomy of what reality is—for example—that there is '*objective reality*' which exists independent of an individual, and that there can also be '*subjective reality*' or '*reality negotiated by groups of people*'. So, the reality of mental health or mental illness could be viewed as something that has always objectively existed independently, or that it can also be viewed as something that did not exist until someone or a group of people subjectively or collaboratively decided what it is.

We see then, that if our epistemology (knowledge of mental health and how we know what we know about it), and our ontology (whether we view the foundation or reality of mental health as something that is objective or subjectively created) can be fundamentally different depending on who we are, our individual or collective experiences and where we come from—then we begin to have a sense of why mental illness can be viewed differently. While you delve into the chapters of this book, if you come across material, or an approach that does not appear to fit with your own understanding it might be helpful to consider or reflect on this with epistemology and ontology in mind. Consider how any differences in perspective may present or inform the area you are reading about. Reflect also on what this might mean for you—for example, if you are a mental health nurse, or a student nurse, consider how differences in views may be manifesting in approaches to understanding or treating psychological distress in the clinical areas you work in. Reflect also on whether this contributes in some way towards enhancing (or not) your day-to-day collaborative approaches to care with individuals who are struggling with their mental health.

HISTORICAL DEVELOPMENTS TO UNDERSTANDING HUMAN DISTRESS AND MENTAL HEALTH NURSING PROGRESSION

Discourse surrounding the history and meaning of psychiatry has been influenced by several works, such as that of Michel Foucault in his 1961 book; *Folie et déraison: Histoire de la folie à l'âge classique*, translated by Richard Howard as '*Madness and Civilization: A History of Insanity in the Age of Reason*'. Bracken (2015) states that although Foucault agreed that psychiatry emerged from a cultural shift of valuing reason and rationality, he also viewed the Age of Reason as detrimental, in effect leading to the massive incarceration of people in the nineteenth and early twentieth century who were seen as *unreasonable* leading to a huge scale of social exclusion.

We briefly explore some key historical characteristics and influences of what was believed to cause mental distress and what was purported to alleviate it. As mentioned earlier in this chapter, we can then begin to reflect on our own thoughts on what may have been helpful or unhelpful aspects; and where this leaves us in contemporary mental health nursing practice. The following is a whistle stop tour of significant practices and developments in 'reacting to' and supporting those experiencing mental distress. Our exploration in this section will be limited to Western health systems and settings, however it is important to acknowledge that mental health care and its evolution over time has occurred at different paces and has been influenced by a variety of factors such as social movements and culture in different countries.

Figure 1.1 provides a brief overview of the key features and events in the historical development of mental health care in the United Kingdom (UK). What is clear from the timeline is that concepts of mental health have been evolving over several centuries. The *Pre 1700s* saw a field that was largely misunderstood, characterised by a sense of hopelessness and it was believed that individuals who were experiencing various forms of distress had no prospects of recovering. They were labelled as lunatics, fools, idiots and imbeciles, and there was a strong view that mood, thought, and behavioural differences were attributed to spirits, gods and demons. Because individuals presented with mood or behaviour that was not considered 'normal' some were feared by their communities and cast out. The approaches to managing those who were mentally

Pre 1700's	1700's	1800's	1900's	2000's
• Individuals with mental illness viewed as different & sometimes considered as possessing wisdom • Individuals with mental illness called fools, lunatics and idiots	• Mental illness attributed to spirits, gods, demons • Theories on morality underpinned societal views • The 'mad' were cast out of society	• Term and feild of 'psychiatry' developed • Rise of lunatic asylums and containment • Lunacy Act (1845) and moral shift to treat individuals with mental illness as patients not prisoners • Stigma recognition	• Compassionate care, closure of asylums & drive for community based care • Human rights informed approaches • Positive influence of the 'Survivor Movement' • Developments in treatment-medication and talking therapies • 1st Edition of the Diagnostic Statistical Manual (DSM)	• Critical perspectives • Strengthening of person centred care • Recognition of trauma and trauma informed approaches in mental health • Development of alternative approaches to diagnosis (Power Threat Meaning Framework [PMTF] & Indicative Trauma Impact Manual [ITIM])

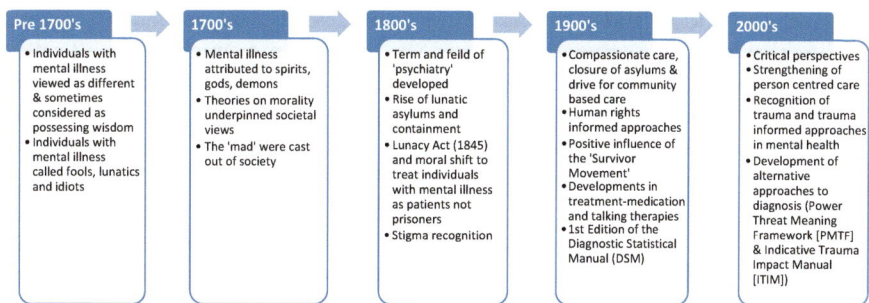

Fig. 1.1 The evolution of mental illness in the UK

ill included imprisonment alongside those who were poor, destitute and offenders. It was common for individuals to be locked in basements, chained to beds, isolated, or even caged to 'manage' 'treat' or 'punish' them. The voices of those who struggled with their mental health were silenced, and not represented in any decisions about what services or care looked like.

There was a shift in the *1800s* following the recognition of a need to provide more appropriate mental health support and treatment. With the recognition that there was scope for development of a branch of medicine specialising in the brain and the mind, the field of Psychiatry was conceived in the 1800s by Johann Reil. While these advances were well meaning, the treatment methods were still of little benefit for those in emotional distress. Interestingly, in addition to the growing view that mental illness was a nervous system dysfunction—advances in civilisation were also viewed as contributors to poor mental health. Moral treatment resurfaced under the Quakers (e.g. The York Retreat in England, UK) characterised by less harm to patients. The 1800s were also marked by a rise in asylums. Asylums were often built to be self-sustaining communities, and it was common for these to have farms and workshops where residents were expected to 'work' and contribute. However, there were still insufficiencies in treatment which included bloodletting, hot and cold baths and patients tied to spinning boards. It is worth noting that although the 1800s saw a rise in asylums, these dated further back to around 1247 where Bethlem Hospital in London was recorded as the 1st Lunatic Asylum in Europe. Moral treatment was viewed as important, and recommendations '*to encourage the influence of religious principles over the mind of the insane [were] considered of great consequence as a means of cure*' (Tuke, 1813). Asylums emerged across other Western countries such as France and Italy (Mora, 1959), and in the United States of America (USA) with the Pennsylvania Lunatic Asylum in 1851. By the middle of the nineteenth century, medical superintendents had gained a monopoly over the treatment of those with mental illness (Scull, 2019).

The *1900s* were considered as a period of growing humane and compassionate approaches to mental health care. Although this had been recognised towards the end of the previous century, the 1900s were particularly pivotal with active civil rights movements, and the survivor movements that all called for fundamental humanistic, compassionate, and ethical care of those who were often disenfranchised (such as those struggling with their mental health, women and people from black and minority ethnic groups). The 1900s also saw the development of the Mental Health Act (1959) which had more recognition of the need for the human rights of those with mental illness to be protected even where the Act itself gave mental health professionals the powers to detain individuals for mental health assessment and or treatment. Developments also included new medications such as antipsychotics (Pillay et al., 2017) and psychotherapies (although from the late 1800s). Perhaps what was most significant about the 1900s was the beginning of the fall of the large asylums as there were calls for a move towards community care, rehabilitation and integration (rather than isolation) of those who struggled with their mental health.

The *2000s* have seen some major leaps in improving mental health care, campaigns on reducing stigma and greater empowerment and advocacy for individuals who are struggling with their mental health. The 2000s have also been characterised by efforts to improve mental health nursing skills, and greater focus on the work of community mental health nurses to support those with severe mental health problems (White & Brooker, 1990). Innovative training such as the Thorn Nurse Programme was introduced to develop mental health nurses' skills in evidence-based psychosocial interventions. As an example, the Thorn Nurse Programme focused upon a stress vulnerability conceptualisation of psychosis and incorporated education on case management, family intervention and the psychological management of psychotic symptoms (O'Carroll et al., 2004; Mairs & Arkle, 2007).

Improving Access to Psychological Therapies (IAPT) was introduced in 2008, with Cognitive Behaviour Therapy (CBT) being focused upon as an evidence-based therapy including associated guidelines recommending CBT-based therapies (NICE, 2004a, 2004b). With these developments, it is known that mental health nurses moved into roles within IAPT services whereby there were professional development opportunities to undertake further training in CBT and to practise in roles such as High Intensity Therapists. The 2000s also began to see the concept of 'recovery' gaining momentum with differentiations proposed between 'clinical recovery' and 'personal recovery'. Clinical recovery has been referred to as the reduction or elimination of symptoms and a returning to a previous state of or improved functioning (Van Eck et al., 2018). A key personal recovery definition has been stated as: '*...a deeply personal, unique process of changing one's attitudes, values, feelings, goals, skills, and/or roles. It is a way of living a satisfying, hopeful, and contributing life even within the limitations caused by illness. Recovery involves the development of new meaning and purpose in one's life as one grows beyond the catastrophic effects of mental illness*' (Anthony, 1993, p. 15).

A narrative review by Leamy et al. (2011) synthesised public descriptions and models of personal recovery into a conceptual framework. The framework consists of thirteen characteristics of the recovery journey and five recovery processes involving the areas of connectedness, hope and optimism about the future, identity, meaning in life and empowerment. These factors are referred to by the acronym CHIME. It is important to note that studies focusing on recovery for individuals from black and ethnic minority groups placed greater emphasis on the areas of spirituality and stigma. Two additional themes were also identified, these being culturally specific facilitating factors and collectivist notions of recovery.

Recovery-focused language has been identified as accurately reflecting an individual's voice to support recovery and does not overly emphasise professionals' opinions (Harris & Felman, 2012). Listening to and supporting an individual to communicate their recovery aims and reflecting this via the language we use to check our understanding is important in supporting those with experiences of mental health problems to move forward in their lives. In a study conducted around mental health stigma, Crisp et al. (2000) advised that it is necessary for practitioners to listen and learn from their patients as people with individual concerns and needs. However, in order to develop sympathetic responses, training and adequate time is required and hence the authors called for adequate staffing in all health and social services.

In integrating those with lived experiences of mental health difficulties into the development and review of services, terminology such as 'service user involvement' was introduced and became more prominent within mental health settings and services. This broad term referred to areas such as participation in service recruitment and interview processes, as well as collaborating on the development of and delivery of care services. Those who used, had used or were carers/family members were invited to be collaborators in service design and reviewing services. 'Service user monitoring' also became a process within many healthcare Trusts. Examples of service user monitoring include contracting experts by experience to spend time on inpatient units, speaking to people who were receiving care to gain feedback on good and problematic aspects of their care or the environment—and then feeding this back to a service representative who could work with the care teams to make improvements if indicated.

We hope that this brief exploration of the historical development of mental health response and support sets the scene and shows how far we have come in mental health, particularly because some of the advances we will explore in the next sections of this chapter are presented as contemporary attempts at addressing the gaps that we still have in mental health care, and mental health nursing skills development.

Multidisciplinary Approaches to Understanding and Responding to an Individual's Distress

Contemporary mental health care involves multidisciplinary teamwork to support those experiencing distress and phenomena affecting behaviour. Members of the mental health multidisciplinary team typically involve the professions of social work, psychiatry, psychology, mental health nursing and allied health professionals, for example occupational therapy. However, recent developments have recognised the importance of re-dressing the power-imbalance within the multidisciplinary team and the 'them and us' organisational setup which promotes a binary position of those without mental health problems and those with. To this end, peer support workers, who have lived experience of mental health difficulties have been introduced into multidisciplinary teams with their support centred on shared experiences, providing empathetic responses and inspiration for recovery to those they are supporting (NHS Health Education England, 2023). Although these are valued roles and demonstrate a more meaningful approach in offering the understanding and therapeutic relationships which may be beneficial for a distressed individual and their family/friends, it does raise a question with regard to how other multidisciplinary members can also demonstrate parity in their experiences of distress and mental health difficulties, so that they too can openly communicate and they may also share some lived experiences of distress themselves. Alec Grant (see Short et al., 2007; Grant, 2016) has brought these issues to the forefront in his autoethnographic writing, especially by requesting that mental health nurses consider reflexive self-disclosure to challenge dominant discourses through reflecting on personal experiences and not becoming 'uncritical culture rule followers' (Grant, 2022).

With a consensus on the importance of cohesive multidisciplinary working and its relationship to high-quality care (Ndoro, 2014), challenges remain in the coordination of care between differing agencies. This is especially pertinent in relation to supporting someone with complex needs within the context of problems spanning both physical and mental health. For further exploration of these issues, see Chap. 4 which outlines how the lack of a coordinated approach can further severely impact on an individual's mental health and support experiences.

Advances in Trauma Informed Approaches: Using the Power Threat Meaning Framework to Formulate Personal Distress

Much of our understanding around mental health has been anchored on the biomedical model which posits that there are biological causes to various mental health conditions, and as such, intervention approaches involve medication to 'treat' the conditions. One of the challenges we face is that in contrast to physical health where there are physical and biological tests that can be done to determine physical ill-health, this is not the case for mental health. One way to illustrate this is using an example of an individual who is diagnosed with diabetes. There are objective scientific ways to do this, such as using the Glycated Haemoglobin (HbA1c) blood test to establish an individual's average blood sugar level over a period of three months. When it comes to diagnosing mental health conditions, we do not have the same physical tests of blood or urine to determine this objectively. There are effectively '*...no biological tests for feeling sad, overwhelmed or angry*' (Thompson & Willets, 2019, p. 161). We do however have self-reporting measures (e.g. questionnaires), but these can be influenced by values, individual judgement, and can be interpreted differently. Thompson and Willets (2019) illustrate using the example of an individual who may have experienced sexual trauma—noting that in the situation where individuals struggle with anxiety and depression, not being able to trust people, their confidence shattered by the experience of sexual trauma—receiving a biomedical 'treatment' of medication is insufficient to tackle the fuller nature of the individual's distress.

It is against this backdrop of debates and controversies that the development of the Power Threat Meaning Framework (PTMF) by Johnstone and Boyle (2018) seeks to contribute to our understanding of mental health and emotional distress. The PTMF aligns well with the global call for a shift towards more human rights underpinned approaches to mental health (Grant & Gadsby, 2018). The PTMF is underpinned by a trauma informed approach, and it encourages a shift from asking 'What's wrong with you? To asking What's happened to you?'. The authors articulate that the PTMF is based on a series of assumptions, namely;

- Emotional distress, unusual experiences and many forms of troubled or troubling behaviour are understandable when viewed in the context of a person's relationships, life events, social circumstances and the standards and expectations we are all expected to live up to.
- There are strong links between personal/family/community distress and social contexts, especially where there is injustice and inequality.
- Different cultural expressions of distress should be accepted and respected.
- We all experience distress at times and the PTMF is about all of us. There is no separate group of people who are 'mentally ill'.
- We all make meaning out of what happens to us, and this shapes the way we experience and express our distress.
- With the right support, we can be active agents in our own lives, rather than seen as victims of medical illness.
- The PTMF gives us tools to create new, hopeful narratives, or stories, about the reasons for our distress that are not based on psychiatric diagnosis. These narratives, which can take many forms, can help us find ways forward as individuals, families, social groups and whole societies. (Boyle & Johnstone, 2020, pp. 3–4)

While the PTMF has been welcomed by many as a contemporary effort to expand our understanding of mental health beyond the biomedical model, it has however been met with some hesitation, criticism and resistance (Boyle & Johnstone, 2020). For example, the very fact that it challenges a dominant way of thinking in mental health (diagnosis) and given that psychiatry has fought hard to be recognised as a legitimate scientific field of medicine, the PTMF is seen by some as a potential threat to the achievements of psychiatry to date. For further reading and exploration of how the PTMF positions itself and identifies the problematic aspects of diagnosis and medicalisation in psychiatry, the fuller document by Johnstone and Boyle (2018) can be accessed online on the British Psychological Society website (BPS, 2024).

ADVANCES IN TRAUMA INFORMED APPROACHES: THE INDICATIVE TRAUMA IMPACT MANUAL (ITIM)

The Indicative Trauma Impact Manual (ITIM) by Taylor and Shrive (2023) presents another contemporary opportunity to advance our understanding of and practice in mental health. Taylor and Shrive present the ITIM as the first non-diagnostic, trauma informed guide to emotion, thought and behaviour, which they have developed with due regard to decades of research, practice experiences, lived experiences and discussions with professionals working with trauma, abuse, and mental health. The ITIM brings into sharp focus issues of oppression, discrimination, misogyny, systemic inequality, and institutions as sometimes simultaneously contributing to trauma, as well as being barriers to trauma informed approaches. It also outlines an example of Anti-Pathologising Trauma Informed Services (APTI) developed as a conceptual approach to support services working in a more trauma informed way by VictimFocus (an international training, research and consultancy organisation working to tackle prejudice and stereotyping of adults and children subjected to crime, violence, abuse and trauma). On a more granular level, the ITIM usefully explores a variety of traumatic experiences—which makes sense, because if we wish to work in a more trauma informed way, there must first be an articulation of what traumatic experiences might include. There might be the perception that major life events such as war, abuse and death are plausible 'traumatic events', however the ITIM explores a wider range of experiences such as how physical illness like anaphylaxis or asthma attacks can be traumatic for some people—impacting to varying degrees an individual's daily life and being the source of pain, panic, fear, helplessness, uncertainty, distress and worry. These examples of trauma experiences serve as useful prompts for professionals to reflect on how people can experience and be affected by trauma—and encourage practitioners to consider what might contribute towards provision of appropriate care.

In a book review, Hughes (2023) highlights that applying a trauma lens to many life experiences in the way Taylor and Shrive have done, shows how distress can manifest in ways that the biomedical model can sometimes overlook. Hughs also adds that if not cautious however, the listing of the trauma experiences may inadvertently replicate the diagnostic nature of the DSM. In some chapters of our book, we begin exploring how the ITIM might be used to connect mental health nursing professional's practice with the perspectives and lived experiences of emotional distress in the individuals they are working with.

Approaches to Formulation

The word 'formulation' can be used in a number of contexts and to refer to a number of processes. These can include psychological formulation and variations to this approach including formulation in the context of risk and safety and to incorporate biological and social aspects.

Psychological Formulation

In psychology and psychotherapy, formulation has been explained as follows:

> *A formulation draws upon psychological theory in order to create a working hypothesis or best guess about the reasons for a client's difficulties, in the light of their relationships and social contexts and the sense they have made of the events in their lives. Formulations are co-constructed with clients, and their main purpose is to inform the intervention.* (Johnstone & Dallos, 2014: preface)

Differing psychological theories can underpin formulation approaches. Here we are outlining key approaches to formulation namely cognitive behavioural therapy (CBT) formulation and psychodynamic formulation as well as touching upon others.

CBT Formulation

CBT formulation is often referred to as 'case formulation' and was seen as a more useful alternative to psychiatric diagnosis as problem behaviour could also be described in terms of environmental factors and responses (Hayes & Follette, 1992; Johnstone & Dallos, 2014). The most prominent and recognised models of CBT approaches of formulation include the 5Ps model (Dudley & Kuyken, 2014) and the 5 areas model (Padesky & Mooney, 1990). The 5Ps of CBT formulation includes an exploration of an individual's presenting issues, precipitating factors, perpetuating factors, predisposing factors and protective factors. An example of a 5Ps formulation is presented in Table 1.1.

The 5Ps approach to formulation can be used to ascertain a contextual picture of a person's presenting problem(s) during the assessment phase of a period of care or treatment. The 5 parts or 5 areas formulation model (Padesky & Mooney, 1990) is a popular way of looking at how our environment or situation may connect to the four aspects of ourselves and how they interlink. These four aspects are: a biological or physical aspect, feelings, behaviour and thoughts. It highlights that if change occurs in one of these areas, then this can impact another area. It can be helpful for people to see that there is a connection between thoughts, feelings, behaviour, biology and environment/situation. It is a model for understanding why changes in thoughts and behaviour can help even problems with biological or environmental factors (Padesky & Mooney, 1990). This type of formulation may also be helpful to identify maintenance cycles—that is factors that keep the problem going (Kennerley et al., 2017). For an example of a 5 areas formulation, see Fig. 1.2.

Table 1.1 An example of a 5Ps formulation based on Dudley and Kuyken's Model (2014)

The 5Ps	*Example of Ellie*
Presenting issues What are the person's presenting emotions, thoughts, behaviours and difficulties?	• Not being able to leave the house • Avoidance of situations • Lack of social networks
Precipitating factors What factors triggered the person's current difficulties and presenting issues?	• Was attacked and mugged on the street • Passersby didn't help and therefore a lack of trust in strangers • Death of mother
Perpetuating factors What are the external and internal factors which continue the person's current difficulties?	• Uses alcohol to 'block things out' • Cancels any plans for social contact • Avoids talking to any remaining friends
Predisposing factors What factors increased the person's vulnerability to their current problems?	• Mother and father had a violent relationship and Ellie used to isolate herself and stay in bedroom • Ellie was frightened of father and has not had many people she trusted whilst growing up
Protective factors What are the person's strengths and resilience that help them maintain their health?	• Can work from home • Plays online games with others • Has two pets • Trusted neighbour visits Ellie, is a friend and gives emotional support

A Psychodynamic Approach to Formulation

Within a psychodynamic approach to formulation is the recognition that the word psychodynamic is used to include the many theoretical approaches interconnected to the roots of psychoanalysis (Leiper, 2014). Psychodynamic formulations should encompass ideas about how unconscious thoughts and feelings may impact the patient's problems and how these unconscious processes may have evolved. It involves delving into a patient's personal history, examining their present problems and patterns, and retracing steps to gain insight into their development. Psychodynamic formulations can explain various aspects of an individual's thoughts, emotions or behaviours. They can be based on a limited amount of information obtained during a single encounter or a comprehensive understanding acquired through long-term analysis. These formulations can account for how an individual behaves in therapy, during specific crises or throughout their lifetime. Psychodynamic formulations are applicable in diverse treatment settings, whether brief or long term, as long as they consider the impact and development of unconscious thoughts and feelings.

The process of constructing a psychodynamic formulation involves three fundamental steps. Firstly, the clinician describes the primary problems and patterns exhibited by the patient, delving beyond surface-level issues to comprehend underlying factors in areas such as self, relationships, adaptation, cognition and work/play. Secondly, a developmental history is reviewed, exploring

Situation:

I sit on the sofa wanting to go to the corner shop.

Thoughts/images:

I imagine seeing a group of teenagers blocking my way.

Physical sensations:

I start feeling hot and can feel my pulse beating quickly. Sometimes I get a sickness feeling.

Emotions:

I feel frightened, panicked, and sad.

Behaviours:

I am glued to the sofa like I can't move. I cover myself up with a blanket.

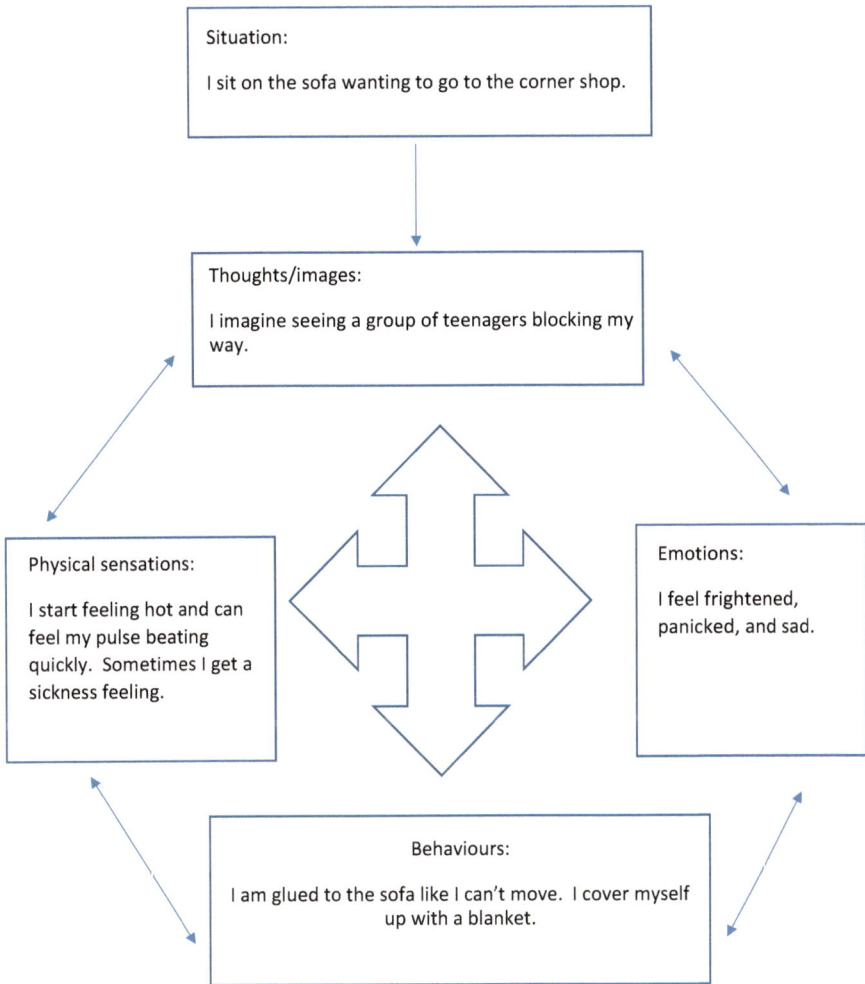

Fig. 1.2 An example of a 5 areas formulation for Ellie

the patient's family background, prenatal development, genetic factors, early relationships, attachment, trauma and subsequent periods of development. This comprehensive understanding encompasses both positive and problematic aspects of their history. Lastly, the clinician establishes connections between the patient's problems and patterns and their developmental history, utilising organising ideas about development. These organising ideas serve as frameworks for conceptualising and understanding how the patient's experiences have influenced their current thoughts, emotions and behaviours. Examples of organising ideas include trauma, early cognitive and emotional difficulties, conflict and defence mechanisms, relationships, self-development and attachment. For an example of applying psychodynamic principles to a formulation, please see Chap. 5.

The Biopsychosocial Model and Formulation

In psychiatry, a biopsychosocial model of case formulation has been developed (see PsychDB, 2024). In this model, the language focuses primarily on a medical underpinning but incorporates biological, psychological and social factors to understand a 'patient' and to guide 'treatment and prognosis'. This approach is based upon the biopsychosocial model, originally described by Engel (1977) and has been said to be a means of understanding a patient as more than a diagnostic label. It explores genetic, personality, psychological factors, biological factors, environmental factors, social circumstances including childhood experiences/adverse events and social determinants of health (SDOH). SDOH can be broken down in to five areas, these being; economic stability, education access and quality, healthcare access and quality, neighbourhood and built environment, and social and community context. For further discussion on aspects of SDOH, see the narrative review of preventative interventions to mental ill-health by Arango et al. (2018). This review highlights that vulnerability trajectories indicate that change is possible at many points during an individual's development. The authors highlight this recognition is important for acting on possibilities for influencing developmental processes towards less debilitating mental health conditions and intervening to support people who may be showing risk factors that can lead to severe disorders in adulthood.

The Recognition of Diversity, Marginalised Groups, Service User Empowerment and Experts by Experience

Historical exploration of how society and systems of power have responded to people with mental health problems demonstrates issues of inequality. There are many examples of this, but in particular the prominent examples which come to mind are the differences in treatment which have occurred for those from a black and ethnic minority background, women—the judgement of women and their behaviour, and those with individual differences which do not fit into a mainstream culture or dominant view of what is 'normal and acceptable' within an historical period and/or political system. Throughout this book, within exploring formulation approaches, some of these issues will be highlighted and explored with regard to the impact this has had on the individual experiencing distress.

However, consulting service users on the planning, evaluation of service quality and providing better health emerged in policy documents associated with the concept of *user involvement* (Department of Health (DoH), 1990, 1991, 1992) with an intention of *partnership working* between service user groups and mental health services. Rush (2004) in their review of user involvement, indicated in stark contrast to partnership approaches, the twenty-first century has brought a spotlight of *risk* and *risk to the general public* which muddies the waters with regard to what extent *user involvement* and *partnership* can be attained. Themes and issues of risk and safety will be drawn upon throughout this book and how in the formulation process, this can be addressed.

We feel it is important to close this section by acknowledging the individuals who have challenged power dynamics within the delivery of mental health services, perceptions of distress and recovery, and service responses to people experiencing behaviours not in keeping with perceptions of 'normality'. These individuals were addressing these issues often long before terms such as 'user involvement' and 'user focussed monitoring' came in to play. Naming a few highly influential individuals who offered critical exploration and challenge to the accepted status quo of outlooks in mental health, we would like to point you in the direction of Ron Coleman, his wife Karen Taylor and Pat Deegan. Ron Coleman has been instrumental in exploring the experience and perceptions of psychosis and hearing voices and concepts of recovery (Coleman, 2011). Karen Taylor has offered a very helpful perspective and support to practitioners in exploring recovery and Ron and Karen's video work are extremely helpful online resources for both students and practitioners in exploring recovery and voice hearing considerations. More recently Ron has focussed upon the exploration of his deterioration in memory (Coleman, 2018).

Pat Deegan is a disability rights advocate, psychologist and researcher. In addition, she has focussed upon supporting individuals and organisations in developing peer support and recovery approaches. She was diagnosed with schizophrenia as a teenager and her long list of publications, conference presentations as well as training events demonstrate innovation and a drive in seeing people as people, rather than focusing on a label or diagnosis. Of course, there are many other inspirational people we could mention in this section and with regard to the survivor movement, but we have started with Ron, Karen and Pat as they have been instrumental in our teachings and lectures within the student populations we have been involved with.

THE CONTRIBUTIONS THAT MENTAL HEALTH NURSING CAN MAKE

As outlined in previous sections, there are many theoretical, lived experience and research-based approaches which can support with exploring the origins and influences of an individual's experiences of distress and/or problematic behaviour. These considerations are important for knowledge building, awareness and for applying in collaborative discussion with the individual we are supporting. But the aims at a foundation stage of providing support possibly led us to exploring the following considerations before leaping in with theories and direct discussion. We would advocate considering the following:

- Have you checked with the individual whether they want to or feel ready to embark on an exploration of their distress? Has this come from the individual themselves?

- Have you transparently explained your views on 'formulation' and sought feedback and questions from the individual you are working with and what they would find helpful?
- Importantly, have you ascertained where you are in the therapeutic relationship process with the individual? Are you gently beginning to build a rapport and trust? Are you very much at the listening stage whereby this may be the most important step throughout the whole journey of supporting the individual; assisting them to feel validated and cared for within the relationship with tentative discussion of their experiences?

The above are broad considerations but important ones for demonstrating the intentions of a genuine and trusting relationship. Outlooks in mental health nursing have focused upon the therapeutic and enabling relationship between nurse and service user (Reed & Hall, 2018). The mental health nurse as a compassionate supporter and helper has been at the centre of discussions regarding the key qualities of what a nurse should demonstrate (Moone & Trenoweth, 2018; Frances Report, 2010). The notion of compassion in nursing is what is most often brought to mind when a person thinks of a nurse and their discerning qualities, but importantly there is a critical perspective here that proposes that the act of compassion can be as instrumental in promoting wellbeing, as much as an intervention in the form of a specific therapy, such as CBT. However, is compassion valued and recognised in its importance as a facilitator of wellbeing as much as a specific therapy? (We note here that there is now 'compassion focussed therapy' and question has compassion been turned in to a therapy to validate its 'effectiveness' and prove its worth via an 'evidence base'?) Do we value and promote the quality of compassion enough in contemporary (mental health) nursing within our daily therapeutic work? We point you to a quote here which may be familiar or not, but once heard it can never be forgotten. Variations of it have been attributed to both the American writer, poet and activist Maya Angelou and Carl W. Buehner, a high-level official in the Mormon church:

> *I've learned that people will forget what you said, people will forget what you did, but people will never forget how you made them feel.*

This quote embodies the notion of connection to an individual with regard to positive feelings enabled by presence and some kind of therapeutic interaction. Carrying the memory and feeling of how an interaction made you feel is important for future contact, interactions and outlooks on spending any amount of time with someone. Feeling included, listened to, respected and validated importantly enhances the experiences of our interactions and being able to display our intentions of striving for these aims is often intertwined with showing and receiving compassion. General definitions of compassion have been associated with pity, sympathy and understanding for someone who is suffering (Collins, 2024).

Within nursing, the professional body in the UK, the Nursing and Midwifery Council (NMC) in its first standard of 'Prioritise People' states that nurses should: 'treat people with kindness, respect and compassion' (NMC, 2015). In addition, The King's Fund (2020) has called to action all health and social care leaders to lead with compassion in addressing the outcomes of a research project which revealed the chronic work pressures which were/are impacting on the delivery of compassionate high-quality care. Although it would appear the notion of compassion is valued and held as a central tenet within nursing practice and nursing leadership, there still remains a vagueness and lack of explicit statements in how compassion underpins not just a values-based approach to supporting others, but how it is a central pivot in a mental health nurse's therapeutic communication to supporting an individual's journey to better mental health. In their exploration of the relevance of compassion to recovery-focused mental health services, Spandler and Stickley (2011, p. 562) highlight the importance of relationship factors (as seen in psychotherapy research) with regard to predictors of positive outcomes rather than a focus upon 'best techniques' or the 'specific model espoused'. They conclude that compassion should be viewed as not just an individual expression, but something which requires nurturing via relationships, cultures and healing environments. Research investigating mental health nurses' views of compassion has highlighted their perceptions of compassionate practice as an emotional response and powerful driver of the provision of relationship-based care (Barron et al., 2017). So where do these considerations of compassion fit when incorporating compassionate mental health nursing practice into collaborative therapeutic formulation? These considerations will begin to be explored in Chap. 2 when we examine both student mental nurses' views and experiences in using formulation, as well as underpinning literature. What we can state here as supporting knowledge, is that compassion needs to be demonstrated as a component of building the therapeutic relationship and establishing a therapeutic alliance between nurse and distressed individual, whereby there is a clear aim and intention by the helper to support someone through an exploration of their distress and engagement within a journey of finding out what may help (Peplau, 1965).

So what opportunities are there for enhancing support for mental health and wellbeing through mental health nurses taking part in formulation? In the UK, the Shape of Caring Review (Health Education England, 2015) outlined the need for undergraduate nursing courses to have greater acquisition of skills that were previously considered advanced or postgraduate—thus creating capacity for the nursing workforce to respond to the complex changing needs of patients more effectively. For mental health nursing, complex clinical work includes developing skills in talking therapies such as cognitive behavioural therapy (CBT), solution focused therapy and learning to use 'formulation' as a skill that is central to the practice of these therapies (Rainforth & Laurenson, 2014). To give an example of the potential capacity that can be harnessed from the mental health nursing workforce alone—20% of mental health nurses in the

UK and 28% of nurses in the USA use CBT, and 12% in the UK and 28% in the USA use an eclectic mix of psychotherapeutic approaches to care (Nolan et al., 2007). NHS England (2023) state the current shortfall in mental health nursing in the UK is a cause for concern, with the greatest vacancy rates in inpatient services, impacting on patient safety and quality of care. They advise that the total mental health nursing shortfall will reach 15,800 FTEs (full-time equivalents) in 2036/37 and point to this being due to fewer nurses taking up training and education and limited opportunities to fill the domestic shortfall with international recruitment. Estimates for required increases in training for mental health nursing are 74–93%. NHS England (2023) state an ambition is to increase training places for mental health nursing by 93% to more than 11,000 places by 2031/32. To support this ambition, by 2028/29 there is an aim to increase training places by 38% for mental health nursing. Identifying transforming agendas in mental health nursing and what will make this a further rewarding and appealing profession could impact on the recruitment and retention of mental health nurses. Enhancing the therapeutic role of the mental health nurse, to recognise more formal psychologically informed approaches, will enable increased training in formulation therefore increasing capacity for skills development, enhancing mental health nursing practice, and more importantly improving support for individuals experiencing challenges with their mental health.

CHAPTER SUMMARY

The introduction chapter has hopefully provided a glimpse of the myriad of understandings of mental health and how formulation can pull together what we know, and support practitioners and patients to work collaboratively towards addressing emotional distress and supporting recovery. The chapter has touched upon the role and relevance of formulation in mental health support and provided an exploration of how mental health nurses (amongst other professionals working in mental health care) can enhance their practice by embracing the principles and practice of formulation (and recovery-focused principles). We will explore more about individual experiences and how formulation may be considered in the various chapters of this book, as well as how we might work with existing approaches to care, while also embracing the more contemporary approaches that support trauma informed practice (such as the PTMF and the ITIM). It is important to note that in the examples used by the upcoming chapter authors, we are not suggesting that there is a 'one size fits all' formulation—but rather, that the principles of formulation are embraced alongside flexibility to work with different models, approaches and lenses to enhance collaborative working. The ultimate goal for considering formulation and the diversity of perspectives and approaches to mental health is to enable us to better support recovery for individuals who are struggling with their mental health. We invite you to use the book as a prompt for critical discussion about the various approaches to supporting and enhancing mental health, and as a guide to reflect on your own position, knowledge and thoughts about where you think the gaps remain. We hope you can draw on the information you find helpful for supporting your decision making and approach to collaborative care planning and care provision.

Points for Reflection

1. Having explored the concepts of epistemology and ontology in this introduction—take a moment to reflect on what your own views are about mental health, and how you have come to know or understand what mental illness is. Make a note of this somewhere and come back to it as you read the chapters of the book.
2. Make a note of what terminology you prefer/tend to use regarding mental health. For example, do you prefer to use the term 'mental illness' or 'emotional distress' or 'mental health disorder' or another term? Then pause to reflect on why you prefer that terminology, and what has influenced your view on this.
3. Having read through the current chapter, reflect on which formulation approach you align with the most, and make a note of why that approach appeals to you.

Organisation of the Remaining Chapters of the Book

Further chapters of the book will draw upon and explore in greater detail some of the underpinning theory and research which has been presented in this introductory opening chapter which has outlined concepts which can facilitate and interlink to formulation within mental health nursing practice. We hope the above areas we have indicated for reflection will be helpful as you navigate your way through the chapters of this book. Below is an overview of each chapter:

Chapter 1—Introduction: Understanding Human Distress and an Invitation to Explore the Myriads of Formulation (this chapter)

Chapter 2—Perspectives on Formulation Within Current Mental Health Nursing Practice

Chapter 3—Three Functions of Using Psychoanalytic and Systemically Informed Perspectives in Case Formulation: Ways of Thinking About Distress in Others, Our Own Reflexivity and Collaborative Formulation

Chapter 4—Formulating Distress in Adults and Children Experiencing Physical and Mental Health Problems

Chapter 5—Formulating Interpersonal Conflict, Relationship Factors and Abuse

Chapter 6—Formulation Considerations for Individuals Experiencing Emotional Distress and Substance Use

Chapter 7—Formulation to Support Individuals Who Are Experiencing Emotional Distress and Associated Self-Harm

Chapter 8—Practitioner Reflections of the Use of Formulation in Mental Health Nursing Practice

Chapter 9—Postscript

REFERENCES

Anthony, W. (1993). Recovery from mental illness: The guiding vision of the mental health service system in the 1990s. *Psychosocial Rehabilitation Journal, 16*, 11–23. https://doi.org/10.1037/h0095655

Arango, C., et al. (2018). Preventative strategies for mental health. *The Lancet; Psychiatry, 5*(7), 591–604.

Barron, K., Deery, R., & Sloan, G. (2017). Community mental health nurses' and compassion: An interpretative approach. *J. Psychiatr. Ment. Health Nurs., 24*, 211–220. https://doi.org/10.1111/jpm.12379

Bochner, A., & Ellis, C. (2016). *Evocative autoethnography*. Routledge.

Boyle, M., & Johnstone, L. (2020). *The power threat meaning framework*. PCCS.

BPS. (2024). Power Threat Meaning Framework (PTMF). https://www.bps.org.uk/member-networks/division-clinical-psychology/power-threat-meaning-framework

Brabazon, T. (2023). *The three wise monkeys of research: Epistemology, ontology and methodology*. Author's Republic.

Bracken, P. (2015). On madness and civilisation: A history of insanity in the age of reason (1961), by Michel Foucault. *The British Journal of Psychiatry., 207*(5), 434–434. https://doi.org/10.1192/bjp.bp.115.165274

Chessler, P. (2018). *Women and madness*. Lawrence Hill Books.

Coleman, R. (2011). *Recovery: An alien concept?* P & P Press.

Coleman, R. (2018). *Dementing disgracefully: Book one the dementia diaries*. CreateSpace Independent Publishing Platform.

Collins Dictionary. (2024). https://www.collinsdictionary.com/dictionary/english/compassion; https://www.collinsdictionary.com/dictionary/english/compassion

Crisp, A. H., Gelder, M. G., Rix, S., Meltzer, H. I., & Rowlands, O. J. (2000). Stigmatisation of people with mental illnesses. *British Journal of Psychiatry, 177*(1), 4–7. https://doi.org/10.1192/bjp.177.1.4

Crotty, M. (1998). *Foundations of social research: Meaning and perspective in the research process* (1st ed.). Routledge.

Crowe, M., Carlyle, D., & Farmar, R. (2008). Clinical formulation for mental health nursing practice. *Journal of Psychiatric and Mental Health Nursing, 15*(10), 800–807. https://doi.org/10.1111/j.1365-2850.2008.01307.x

Department of Health (DoH). (1990). *The NHS and Community Act*. HMSO.

Department of Health (DoH). (1991). *The Patients Charter*. HMSO.

Department of Health (DoH). (1992). *The health of the nation*. HMSO.

Dudley, R., & Kuyken, W. (2014). Case formulation in cognitive behavioural therapy: A principle driven approach. In L. Johnstone & R. Dallos (Eds.), *Formulation in psychology and psychotherapy: Making sense of people's problems* (2nd ed., pp. 18–44). Routledge.

Eghigian, G. (2019). *The Routledge history of madness and mental health*. Routledge.

Ellis, C. (2017). Manifesting compassionate autoethnographic research: Focusing on others. *International Review of Qualitative Research, 10*(1). https://doi.org/10.1525/irqr.2017.10.1.54

Engel, G. (1977). The need for a new medical model: A challenge for biomedicine. *Science, 196,* 129–136. https://doi.org/10.1126/science.847460

Foucault, M. (1961). *Déraison et folie: Histoire de la folie à l'âge classique.* Paris: Plon.

Frances Report. (2010). *Report of the Mid Staffordshire NHS Foundation Trust public inquiry: Executive summary.* Crown.

Grant, A. (2016). Living my narrative: Storying dishonesty and deception in mental health nursing. *Nurs Philos, 17,* 194–201. https://doi.org/10.1111/nup.12127

Grant, A. (2022). What has autoethnography got to offer mental health nursing? *British Journal of Mental Health Nursing,* 11(4), 4–11. https://doi.org/10.12968/bjmh.2022.0035

Grant, A., & Gadsby, J. (2018, September). The Power Threat Meaning Framework and international mental health nurse education: A welcome revolution in human rights. *Nurse Educ Today, 68,* 1–3. https://doi.org/10.1016/j.nedt.2018.05.007. Epub 2018 May 21. PMID: 29864711.

Harris, J., & Felman, K. (2012). *A guide to the use of recovery-oriented language in service planning, documentation, and correspondence.* Mental Health America Allegheny County. Retrieved from chrome-extension://efaidnbmnnnibpcajpcglclefindmkaj/; https://assets.website-files.com/5a13853ae83c4100019201c8/5fd91448e81d68 5e8729a58a_Recovery-Oriented%20Language.pdf

Hayes, S., & Follette, W. (1992). Can functional analysis provide a substitute for syndromal classification? *Behavioural Assessment., 14*(3), 345–365.

Health Education England. (2015). *Raising the bar shape of caring: A review of the future education and training of registered nurses and care assistants.* Health Education England.

Hughes, Y. (2023). Book review: Indicative trauma impact manual. *Psychosis, 15*(4), 424–425. https://doi.org/10.1080/17522439.2023.2233604

Jennings, B., & Loan, L. (2001). Misconceptions among nurses about evidence based practice. *Journal of Nursing Scholarship, 33*(2), 121–127.

Johnstone, L., & Boyle, M. (2018). *The power threat meaning framework: Towards the identification of patterns in emotional distress, unusual experiences and troubled or troubling behaviour, as an alternative to functional psychiatric diagnosis.* British Psychological Society.

Johnstone, L., & Dallos, R. (2014). *Formulation in psychology and psychotherapy making sense of people's problems.* Routledge.

Kennerley, H., Kirk, J., & Westbrook, D. (2017). *An introduction to cognitive behaviour therapy.* SAGE.

Leamy, M., Bird, V., Le Boutillier, C., Williams, J., & Slade, M. (2011). Conceptual framework for personal recovery in mental health: systematic review and narrative synthesis. *The British Journal of Psychiatry, 199*(6), 445–452. https://doi.org/10.1192/bjp.bp.110.083733

Leiper, R. (2014). Psychodynamic formulation: Looking beneath the surface. In L. Johnstone & R. Dallos (Eds.), *Formulation in psychology and psychotherapy: Making sense of people's problems* (pp. 45–66). Routledge.

Mairs, H., & Arkle, N. (2007). *Accredited training in psychosocial interventions for psychosis: a national survey.* NIMHE.

Moone, N., & Trenoweth, S. (2018). Mental health assessment. In K. Wright & M. McKeown (Eds.), *Essentials of mental health nursing* (pp. 329–340). Sage.

Mora, G. (1959). Vincenzo Chiarugi (1759–1820) and his psychiatric reform in Florence in the 18th century. *Journal of the History of Medicine and the Allied Health Sciences, 14*, 424–433.

Ndoro, S. (2014). Effective multidisciplinary working: The key to high-quality care. *British Journal of Nursing, 23*(13), 724–727.

NHS England. (2023). *NHS long term workforce plan.* NHS England.

NHS Health Education England. (2022). *Commitment and growth: Advancing mental health nursing now and for the future.* HEE.

NHS Health Education England. (2023, October 6). *Supporting the individual's well-being, giving hope and supporting recovery.* Retrieved from Health Education England: https://www.hee.nhs.uk/our-work/mental-health/new-roles-mental-health/peer-support-workers

NICE. (2004a). *Anxiety: Management of anxiety (panic disorder, with and without agoraphobia, and generalised anxiety disorder) in adults in primary, secondary and community care. Clinical guideline 22.* National Institute for Health and Clinical Excellence.

NICE. (2004b). *Depression:Management of depression in primary and secondary care. Clinical guideline 23.* National Institute for Health and Clinical Excellence.

NMC. (2015). *The code: Professional standards of practice and behaviour for nurses, midwives and nursing associates.* NMC.

Nolan, P., Haque, S., & Doranc, M. (2007). A comparative cross-sectional questionnaire survey of the work of UK and US mental health nurses. *International Journal of Nursing Studies, 44*, 377–385.

O'Carroll, M., Rayner, L., & Young, N. (2004). Education and training in psychosocial interventions: A survey of Thorn Initiative course leaders. *Journal of Psychiatric and Mental Health Nursing, 11*, 602–607.

Padesky, C., & Mooney, K. (1990). Clinical tip: Presenting the cognitive model to clients. *International Cognitive Therapy Newsletter, 6*(1), 13–14.

Peplau, H. (1965, February). *Interpersonal relationships in nursing.* Paper presented at Council on Hospital Services Institute, District of Columbia-Delaware Hospital Association. Washington DC.

Pillay, J., Boylan, K., Carrey, N., Newton, A., Vandermeer, B., Nuspl, M., … Hartling, L. (2017). *First- and second-generation antipsychotics in children and young adults: Systematic review update.* Agency for Healthcare Research and Quality (US); (Comparative Effectiveness Reviews, No. 184.).

PsychDB. (2024). Biopsychosocial model and case formulation. https://www.psychdb.com/teaching/biopsychosocial-case-formulation

Rainforth, M., & Laurenson, M. (2014). A literature review of case formulation to inform mental health practice. *Journal of Psychiatric and Mental Health Nursing, 21*(3), 206–213. https://doi.org/10.1111/jpm.12069

Reed, M., & Hall, S. (2018). Therapeutic engagement for mental health care. In K. Wright & M. McKeon (Eds.), *Essentials of mental health nursing* (pp. 314–327). Sage.

Rush, B. (2004). Mental health service user involvement in England: Lessons from history. *Journal of Psychiatric and Mental Health Nursing, 11*, 313–318.

Scull, A. (2019). The asylum, hospital, and clinic. In G. Eghigian (Ed.), *The Routledge history of madness and mental health* (pp. 101–114). Routledge.

Short, N., Grant, A., & Clarke, L. (2007). Living in the borderlands; Writing in the margins: An autoethnographic tale. *Journal of Psychiatric and Ment Health Nursing, 14*, 771–782. https://doi.org/10.1111/j.1365-2850.2007.01172.x

Shorter, E. (1997). *A history of psychiatry: From the Era of the Asylum to the Age of Prozac.* John Wiley & Sons.

Spandler, H., & Stickley, T. (2011). No hope without compassion: The importance of compassion in recovery-focused mental health services. *The Journal of Mental Health, 20*(6), 555–566. https://doi.org/10.3109/09638237.2011.583949

Taylor, J., & Shrive, J. (2023). *Indicative trauma impact manual: A non-diagnostic, trauma-informed guide to emotion, thought, and behaviour* (1st ed.). VictimFocus.

The King's Fund. (2020). The courage of compassion: Supporting nurses and midwives to deliver high quality care. https://www.kingsfund.org.uk/sites/default/files/2020-09/The%20courage%20of%20compassion%20summary_web_0.pdf https://www.kingsfund.org.uk/sites/default/files/2020-09/The%20courage%20of%20compassion%20summary_web_0.pdf

Thompson, L., & Willets, B. (2019). Towards a trauma informed approach with people who have experienced sexual violence. In J. Watson (Ed.), *Drop the disorder: Challenging the culture of psychiatric diagnosis* (pp. 160–167). PCCS Books.

Titler, M. (2006). *Developing an evidence-based practice* (6th ed.). Mosby.

Tuke, S. (1813). *Description of the retreat.* Society of Friends.

Van Eck, R., Burger, T., Vellinga, A., Schirmbeck, F., & de Haan, L. (2018). The relationship between clinical and personal recovery in patients with schizophrenia spectrum disorders: A systematic review and meta-analysis. *Schizophrenia Bulletin, 44*(3), 631–642. https://doi.org/10.1093/schbul/sbx088

White, E., & Brooker, C. (1990). The future of community psychiatric nursing: What might the Care Programme Approach mean for practice and education? *Community Psychiatric Nursing Journal, 10*(6), 27–30.

CHAPTER 2

Perspectives on Formulation Within Current Mental Health Nursing Practice

Vickie Howard and Lolita Alfred

> **Key Learning Points**
> - An exploration of the literature on formulation in mental health nursing
> - Engaging learners—mental health nursing student perspectives on formulation
> - Exploring a family member's experiences of approaches to treatment and professional decision making
> - A summary of identified issues on formulation from this chapter

This chapter will draw together some of the current considerations around using formulation within mental health nursing practice. It will begin by identifying the literature currently available to us which involves mental health nursing professionals as part of the multidisciplinary team who use and contribute to formulation, whether this be individually or as part of a team. We will then move on to examining student mental health nursing views and perspectives on using formulation by presenting outcomes from two online activities which were part of a module on learning about formulation in both undergraduate and postgraduate programmes. We will close the chapter with what all this may mean for the current use, development of and future outlooks on

V. Howard (✉)
Faculty of Health Sciences, University of Hull, Hull, UK
e-mail: V.Howard@Hull.ac.uk

L. Alfred
City, University of London, London, UK
e-mail: Lolita.Alfred@city.ac.uk

© The Author(s), under exclusive license to Springer Nature Switzerland AG 2024
V. Howard, L. Alfred (eds.), *Formulation in Mental Health Nursing*, https://doi.org/10.1007/978-3-031-59956-9_2

what formulation could look like, which will lead in to the 'doing collaborative formulation' chapters of the book. In these chapters, different authors and contributors demonstrate their outlooks, practical applications and use of formulation—with the aim of helping an individual reflect on wellbeing factors.

Using Formulation Within Mental Health Nursing Practice: What the Literature Says

The use of formulation within mental health practice has been explored and evidenced from its use by psychologists. This makes sense when considering that formulation is a core competency of the role of clinical psychologists as it underpins psychological intervention (British Psychological Society, 2010). The prevalence of models of formulation appear to mainly centre around a cognitive behavioural therapy (CBT) approach, whereby the 5P model has been used to link presenting problems to predisposing, precipitating, perpetuating and protective factors. A study by McTiernan et al. (2021) found that using the 5P approach within team formulation functioned as a cognitive learning process that facilitated a deeper knowledge and understanding of clients. Three nursing staff were involved in this study which comprised of individual interviews of six multidisciplinary staff from a psychosis rehabilitation unit. This study highlights key considerations in the use of team formulation including its ability to reinforce team support and team working. It also raised questions about whether closed staff forums enabling staff discussion as in this study, are preferable to involving clients because they allow this focused staff space for exploration. Concerns about distressing some clients and their psychological vulnerability were voiced by some staff and formulation was viewed as a step from the biomedical model and a move towards a more biopsychosocial process. Hartley's (2021, p. 4) discussion on team formulation expands on the issues of formulation as a collaborative process between mental health professional and service user and she states that *"formulation should always seek to meaningfully involve the client—either in person or in the form of their perspective, views, concerns and wishes."* This article is helpful in presenting how individual team members may be involved in team formulation and contribute according to their role and relationship with the service user. It is a continuing professional development (CPD) article and as such gives mental health nurses ideas on how team formulation may be developed in their practice. The article also points out key considerations including how formulation may also impact on staff members emotionally and cause some areas of discomfort which may require supportive reflection. In addition, it points out that power imbalances are inherent in the mental health system and some service users may experience formulation as harmful and as such informed consent and how information is used should be explicitly stated. Again, this article illustrates the 5Ps model of formulation as an effective starting point for structuring information towards a shared understanding and to generate ideas for future support and therapeutic interventions.

A further CPD article by Cox (2020) focussing upon the implementation of individual formulation presents both the 5Ps model and 5 areas model. The 5 areas model (Williams & Chellingsworth, 2010) is identified as a means of providing a whole-person biopsychosocial assessment to understand a person's presenting problems and works towards using CBT principles to change unhelpful thoughts and behaviours to enable clear targets for change. This publication particularly identifies barriers and solutions to formulation approaches, especially in consideration for the mental health nurse's role. One issue highlighted is that of who takes responsibility for formulation as it is stated that formulation is often seen as the role of the psychologist rather than mental health nurses. It is also stated that research and training for mental health nurses on using formulation is limited and that supervision and support systems should be in place to support the application of skills and interventions.

An article by Yeandle et al. (2015) considers the complexities of 'personality disorders' when aiming to work collaboratively with individuals who may find trusting and maintaining interpersonal relationships very difficult. They highlight the centrality of interpersonal relationships to mental health nursing citing both Peplau (1952) and Barker (2001) in their progression of the notion of the importance of collaborative engagement, assessment and intervention with the distressed person and developing co-constructed narratives. Yeandle et al. (2015) particularly highlight a guided formulation approach which incorporates the recognition of early experiences with current patterns of relating and how this affects feelings, behaviours and relationships leading to shared understanding and further supportive treatment options. Working concurrently with the guided formulation is a key aim of supporting the individual to recognise their strengths, developing ways to reduce distress and negate the need for mental health service intervention.

Clark and Clarke (2014) bring in a further dimension when considering the use of the biopsychosocial approach within 'psychiatric nursing' which would usually just focus upon the biological, psychological and social factors to assess an individual's needs and would be used to plan associated interventions. The biopsychopharmasocial approach (BPPS) advocated by Clark and Clarke (2014) introduces a pharmacological domain to recognise the wider role that pharmaceuticals may have in an individual's daily life. This translates to the presentation of the BPPS matrix with the intention of providing a multiperspective model of formulation that is developed chronologically. The matrix includes an exploration of the following factors; predisposing, precipitating, perpetuating and protective leading to a range of possible identifying interventions with the authors suggesting that an integrated care plan may focus upon psychiatric medication, skills and vocational training, relationship counselling, substance misuse harm reduction, peer-group support work and network support. This article also highlights the importance of recognising the possibility of *diagnostic overshadowing* which is a term describing physical symptoms being misattributed to mental health problems and distress (Jones et al., 2008). This is an important concept to consider and relates to formulation with regard to clinical decision making and the communication which is occurring between the professional and patient. It is especially pertinent considering that those with 'mental illness' die prematurely and experience significantly higher medical co-morbidity than those in the general population (Harris & Barraclough, 1998).

Critical Points for Inquiry from the Literature

In reviewing this literature regarding using formulation within mental health nursing practice, particular themes and points have been highlighted for us as chapter authors. We discuss these below but encourage you to consider what stood out for you and any questions which you may now have regarding the implications of using formulation in mental health nursing practice.

Being Explicit on the Purpose of the Formulation: Who Is It For?

The literature we have sourced has encouraged us to reflect on being explicit on the purpose of the formulation and gain the service user's outlook and view on whether this may be helpful for them in exploring their current difficulties. This would be with an aim of understanding influencing factors—in order to move forward with potentially helpful approaches that would support their wellbeing in the future. The issue of informed consent was raised and the potential for formulation to cause distress or unintentional harm and this needs to be a serious consideration. In addition, a number of articles mentioned formulation as a helpful process in ascertaining risk assessment and management processes. Again, we ask, is the service user informed of this or is this a service driven objective/need? Does this move away from the formulation being about the service user's outlooks? In essence, how the information from the formulation will be used and who it will be made available to needs explicit explanation and consent obtained.

Organisational Structure and Support to Enable Mental Health Nurses to Use Formulation

Although some examples in the literature demonstrate how members of the multidisciplinary team, namely psychologists, have promoted inclusive cultures regarding other team members including mental health nurses being involved in formulation, this is not a standardised and widespread way of working. Many of the articles pointed to the importance of supervision and training as imperative to support mental health nurses and other team members in using formulation skills and approaches well, and this requires organisational support and agreed protocols. In addition, expanding on the accessible 5Ps approach via training to incorporate other therapeutic formulation approaches that mental health nurses can support such as the 5 areas model would require additional recognition (from a service perspective) that this would be a valuable therapeutic addition to their skill set.

Where Is the Service User/Distressed Person's Voice?

The literature we have accessed in relation to mental health nursing practice and formulation does not explicitly include a service user/client/patient/person being supported. Chapters within this book incorporate the person being supported, their outlooks, experiences and views about the use of formulation.

Bringing in the Dimension of the Unique Qualities of Mental Health Nurses to Complement Formulation Processes

There is a lack of an exploration in the literature specifically in facets of mental health nurse roles and how differing formulation approaches may or may not fit.

Student Mental Health Nursing Views and Experiences in Using Formulation

To set a foundation enquiry around factors influencing the current use of formulation within mental health nursing practice, we have undertaken a piece of research exploring student mental health nurses' views and experiences in using formulation. It is encouraging to see that there is evidence of the teaching of formulation in mental health nursing curriculums (in the UK) and some inspiring examples of practice and purpose upon which to build. We firstly wanted to explore student mental health nurses' views towards using formulation within their role and in anticipation of becoming registered practitioners and secondly wanted to enquire further about how a student mental health nurse approaches information given about a person's presenting difficulties.

We will begin with our first enquiry/exercise whereby we asked students to read an article by Crowe et al. (2008) on the use of formulation in mental health nursing practice. The article outlines views on how formulation can assist in linking assessment outcomes to nursing interventions in a meaningful way and outlines some formulation approaches including CBT, psychodynamic and interpersonal formulation. You may want to access this article yourself and compare your own answers and thoughts to those of the involved students in this exercise. We set questions on a discussion board of a online virtual learning environment (VLE) and asked the students;

1. Which of the approaches to formulation do you align with and would feel comfortable using?
2. If you were setting up a new mental health service, how would you design it to ensure mental health nurses either take part or lead on formulation in practice?
3. The article was published in 2008 and states that; "there is no literature available on the use of clinical formulation in mental health nursing..." Conduct a quick scoping literature search (e.g. using Google or Google Scholar) and see if you can find any literature or research or general info/

articles on the use of formulation in mental health nursing. If so, either note the reference of the information you find or provide a hyperlink so others can view this … provide a comment on what you think to the information you have found.
4. Comment on at least one other post…

A summary of the results is presented in Table 2.1. The students who participated in the exercises in this chapter included both undergraduate and postgraduate mental health nursing students from two academic higher education institutions. Ethical processes and procedures were followed regarding the application and authorisation of ethics approval from the institutions involved.

What This Exercise Has Demonstrated

Student response numbers showed a preference for the description of interpersonal formulation as a choice in practice, though the reasons behind this are unsubstantiated. We have surmised a possible reason may be student mental health nurses may feel more confident and familiar with the underlying premises of this form of formulation in the absence of training on other specific formulation approaches including CBT and psychodynamic. There was a strong voice in the call for training in formulation approaches to support both individual skills and the idea of team members working together with areas of formulation practice. When attempting to find literature on formulation, students struggled to find a large body of literature and presented the same articles. Although a few articles were found published in 2020 and 2021 these were not research articles—again indicating there is a lack of research to inform formulation practice and development for mental health nurses and students.

The second VLE exercise we set for students involved asking them to read an article titled 'Boy, Interrupted: A Story of Akathisia' (Loomer, 2021). The article, written from a mother's experiences portrays her son's journey in finding answers regarding his mental distress via a range of mental health professionals and trying to piece together what had and what was happening to him. It raises important themes regarding being listened to, placing the distressed person's experiences as central to the discussion (or not) and prescribing medication and the harmful and long-lasting effects it may have. The very authentic and moving manner in which Loomer tells her story is a valuable resource in considering formulation and how an approach incorporating the collaborative formulation we are advocating for in this book, may challenge some of the heavily medicalised and dominant narratives which may underpin Loomer's and her son's experiences. The article has been reproduced with permission from Mad in America and Lisa Loomer and is presented in Fig. 2.1.

You may want to pause for a while here and gather your thoughts about what Lisa Loomer has discussed in this article.

For our second VLE exercise we asked mental health nursing students to read this article too and consider the following questions:

Table 2.1 Mental health nursing student exercise on formulation

Question	A sample of student comments	Analysis and summary
Which of the approaches to formulation do you align with and would feel comfortable using?	"I think I'd feel most comfortable using the cognitive behavioural formulation. In practice, I don't think I'd like to use the psychodynamic formulation because it feels like I'm blaming the service user by saying that they have an inability to cope with situations that other people can…" "I would prefer using the psychodynamic formulation. The patient is actively involved and also reflects on themselves and this could be more helpful when creating a plan of care." "I can see the value in all the approaches which is shown by the fact that the subject of the case study used several approaches to help them to understand and change their ways of thinking. I would probably feel most comfortable with the cognitive behavioural approach but the interpersonal approach is also interesting." "In response to this question, I honestly do not know which one I would use. I think they are all beneficial in some ways but they a so have some areas which I believe are not beneficial. For instance CBT is great but requires the service user to engage in talking and some service users do not feel comfortable with talking therapies. I really like the psychodynamic formulation, but again what if the presenting issues do not relate to childhood? I think I need more experience on using each of these to have more of a professional opinion." "I would use interpersonal formulation because this would include using the strong relationships mental health nurses create with their patients."	In choosing an approach students align to and may feel comfortable using, comments indicate students are assimilating their knowledge but may require more education and practical experience of using formulation in practice. As a whole the interpersonal approach was chosen by most students but often without giving a justification for this. We surmise that mental health nurses identified with the description of interpersonal formulation which they linked to approaches used within their nursing practice which focussed on exploring relationships, links to mental health problems and how in their role the use of the therapeutic relationship is used to facilitate these discussions.

(continued)

Table 2.1 (continued)

Question	A sample of student comments	Analysis and summary
How would you design a mental health service to ensure mental health nurses either took part or lead on formulation in practice?	"I think that education of formulation would be paramount and that all members of the team would need a good understanding of formulation approaches and the importance of them in building therapeutic relationships with all patients in order to be able to plan a patient's care effectively to suit their individual needs. This would include everyone who comes into contact with a patient in order for them to understand the importance of information that is shared with them and how this can facilitate a patient's recovery." "When a patient comes into a mental health service, if this is an acute setting or within the community, their first point of contact is with a mental health nurse, who does the information in which they need to add to this person's file, and to create the care plan whilst they are under their care. It is then the psychologist who intervenes and does the formulation. I feel the nurse who was the first point of contact should be involved within this, and to be able to have their own thoughts and views included. I feel as a whole whoever is included within this patient's care should be entitled to be included within the formulation, so I would make this mandatory if I was to set up a new mental health service." "I think nurses should have more of an input with formulation as they do spend a lot of time with service users, assessing, care planning, engaging etc. Service users may also feel more comfortable having their named nurse more involved with this, as the therapeutic relationship may already be formed. Ideally all involved should have relevant and adequate training." "Multiple training sessions."	Students have identified preparatory components including education and training in formulation. They have also identified features of a mental health nurse's role which would place them in a strong position to be involved or lead on formulation. These include the mental health nurse as information gatherer, assessor and the individual the service user may have already formed a therapeutic relationship with which can be built upon.

Student search for literature/research or general info/ articles on the use of formulation in mental health nursing	"Rainforth and Laurenson (2014) conducted a literature review and found information regarding the need for any mental health practitioner needing a degree of knowledge of psychology in order to be able to formulate care effectively which can be gained through the provision of training. They outlined the need for feedback in the form of supervision, the confusion of whether formulation should be standardised or individualised and concluded that more research is still required in order to identify the efficacy of formulation. Rainforth, M. and Laurenson, M. (2014) A literature review of case formulation to inform mental health practice. Psychiatric and Mental Health Nursing, 21(3), 206–213."	Although some literature was identified by students, they did not identify a wealth of sources.
	"When I searched up till 2008 I couldn't find any, but after there were several https:// onlinelibrary.wiley.com/doi/abs/10.1111/jpm.12069" https://www-magonlinelibrarycom.hull.idm.oclc.org/doi/full/10.12968/ bjmh.2018.7.2.75 (Links to an external site.) This research is about team formulation and concludes people do value this however it also brings to light some barriers to team formulation."	
	"This article is in the mental health practice journal which is funny as I subscribed to this and this article is very recent as 2021, https://journals.rcni.com/mental-health-practice/ cpd/use-of-individual-formulation-in-mental-health-practice-mhp.2020.e1515/full (Links to an external site.) this article is interesting as it links aspects of the NMC code and how these aspects are part of formulation, saying that the skills are there for nurses to do formulation."	
Comments on fellow students' posts	"I agree with regular reflective practice groups. In one of my placements they did this once a week with as many of the MDT as possible. I found it was really beneficial."	There was shared agreement around the benefits on team members and roles sharing formulation.
	"I agree and feel that formulation should be collaborative, with everyone who is in contact with the patient. As information that is shared by the patient may vary depending on who the patient is speaking with and the relationship that they have with that person. Vital information may be missed."	

Boy, Interrupted: A Story of Akathisia

By Lisa Loomer

June 13, 2021, Mad in America

One of the side effects of the Covid epidemic has been a sharp rise in the use of antidepressants and anti-anxiety medication. A Market Watch study back in May of 2020, already showed anti-anxiety drug sales jumping 34.1 percent and a rise in antidepressants at 18.6 percent.

And I get it. To tell you the truth, I'm still feeling a little anxious myself. Maybe just a quarter of a Xanax? Cause this week I go to my local pharmacy to get the vaccine. And I know, why worry, right? Fauci says to get it. Biden says to get it. All my friends have gotten it and are beginning to look at me askance… am I paranoid, unpatriotic, a quack?

Maybe I'm just a little more hesitant about pharmaceuticals these days… even that little peach Xanax… ever since my son's life was irrevocably changed by a medication-induced injury called "akathisia."

When I first heard the word "akathisia," it sounded like one of those Greek goddesses—the goddess Akathisia. Like Athena or Aphrodite, she'd be powerful, fierce, but maybe rather… moody? Well, I've come to know Akathisia intimately now. She is devastating, elusive, cruel beyond belief. And for two years I've been battling her for what I love most in the world. Because Akathisia can take an active, bright, successful, charming, compassionate, twenty-one-year-old, drag him down to the underworld, and make his life a living hell.

But let me step back and talk about akathisia from a calmer perspective. A societal perspective. Because this story is not just personal. It's about America's ongoing proclivity toward antidepressants, and it's about Big Pharma. So, while I count down for my J&J or Moderna or Pfizer, let me tell you a little of our personal story and give you a sense of the larger story as well.

For my son, Marcello, akathisia appeared suddenly in the summer of 2019, after just a few weeks on antidepressants taken for garden-variety anxiety. Unusual? Not really. After all, 13.2 percent of Americans are on antidepressants. For women over a certain age, it's one in four. Antidepressants are the third most prescribed class of drugs in America and an almost sixteen billion-dollar a year industry for the drug companies, who make over twenty-five thousand dollars per second on psychiatric meds.

If you have not taken one yourself, surely you have a friend or family member who has, and it's likely they are doing well. But there is a percentage of people who are effectively poisoned by them. (In the simplest of terms, think of it like a peanut allergy.) The FDA claims it's about five percent. Other sources, such as the Akathisia Alliance, an online research site, say it's more like fifteen percent.

There are many "side effects" listed with antidepressants. Most people toss that little paper with the side effects, just as we ignore the warnings on TV commercials, maybe because if we looked too deeply, we'd never take the pill. But one of the side effects mentioned with antidepressants is

Fig. 2.1   Boy, interrupted: A story of Akathisia by Lisa Loomer

"restlessness." And that's basically what the drug companies are willing to tell us about akathisia, that it's an "inner and outer restlessness."

Google it and you'll also find "anxiety or agitation, feeling bad or depressed, distress and panic, a feeling of wanting to jump out of your skin, dark and unpleasant thoughts, strange and unusual impulses, often of an aggressive nature, homicidality, suicidality."

What the drug companies' warnings are not telling us is that akathisia is not really a side effect at all. It's a whole new condition, a neurological as opposed to a psychiatric condition... caused by the drugs themselves. Akathisia is damage to the brain and to virtually every system in the body. Sometimes, the worst of it begins to subside when meds are discontinued. Often it does not.

Sufferers describe akathisia as "like having your blood replaced with battery acid" or "like being burned alive in a locked coffin." They say it's "like being violently tortured from the inside out." Some psychiatrists will tell a patient their symptoms are "somatic." But there are people with absolutely no history of psychiatric illness who get akathisia from a single shot of Reglan, an anti-nausea drug given in hospital settings.

Historically, akathisia has been intentionally induced as part of chemical warfare. In fact, Hitler himself played around with psych meds—and the quick withdrawal of those meds—as a means of torture. Do I sound like a conspiracy theorist? I'm not. I'm a mother who watched her son's life change almost overnight, as he developed drug toxicity from antidepressants taken as prescribed.

At twenty-one, Marcello was a student at The New School in New York with an interest in climate science and psychology. Interestingly, he now sees akathisia as akin to climate change on the level of the human organism. He recognizes that our bodies were simply not designed to properly deal with the man-made drugs we're putting into them.

While living in New York, he was spending a lot of time at the Hayden Planetarium as he'd always loved astronomy, and in New York, he really missed the stars. As a child in Oregon, he was always getting the neighbors to look up through his telescope in the driveway. He'd had gallery showings of his night sky photography as a teenager.

Now, a sophomore in college, he was asking the questions a lot of young men ask... Who am I, where do I fit in? So, he took his junior year off to think about those questions and travelled all over Europe. And when he returned from the trip of a lifetime, he went to see a psychiatrist because he was feeling kind of anxious about his next move. Of course, a lot of folks were feeling anxious. Trump was elected just as Marcello went off to college in 2016, and the collective diagnosis of "anxiety" in America soared at that time.

Still, in Marcello's circle, his friends seemed to be thriving despite their anxiety... often with the help of antidepressants. His best friend become an overnight multimillionaire at twenty-one by coming up with a financial trading algorithm. He bought a Rolex and began buying a fleet of exotic cars. The American Dream? Big time. He was on Lexapro. Another friend was on Zoloft and thriving in the tech industry. Several friends were on Ritalin and doing great in school.

All his friends knew what they wanted to major in, what they wanted to be, who they wanted to be with. Marcello wasn't so sure. He was diagnosed with "Generalized Anxiety Disorder," the most

Fig. 2.1 (continued)

popular diagnosis in this country, and he was curious to see if meds would help. After all, they seemed to be helping his friends.

When he got to our home in Los Angeles, he started seeing a highly respected psychiatrist, and took Cymbalta for just eight days. On the eighth day, he went camping near Big Sur with his other best friend. Karen is the antithesis of the male best friend with the financial algorithm and the cars. She's a botanist, deeply connected to the natural world.

Marcello and Karen went for a day hike, and he missed a dose of Cymbalta. During their hike, the extreme "restlessness" and "inner terror" appeared for the first time. He recalls that it felt like being "acutely poisoned", along with full body pain and vertigo. He thought he'd picked up some kind of insect bite on the trail.

They went to the nearest ER, where he was misdiagnosed with "heat exhaustion." In hindsight, we know that he was experiencing a catastrophic reaction to the drug—a literal poisoning. Back then, we had no idea.

His psychiatrist switched him from Cymbalta to Prozac. He took it for two weeks. One night, after a slight dosage increase, he felt that same powerful inner restlessness—and a brand new kind of anxiety that was a thousand times greater than anything he'd experienced before. He couldn't stay still.

We called his psychiatrist, who said, "Gee… this sounds like akathisia!" She pulled him off Prozac and prescribed Xanax, which, we now know, masks the symptoms of akathisia in the short term. He took Xanax for two and a half months, during which he embarked on a backpacking trip with friends near Mount Rainier in Washington. But he couldn't do it. He wound up sleeping in his car instead of under the stars. He felt terrified, and physically, just really off. He came home to L.A.

Something was different and very wrong. He couldn't go back to school in New York. He wanted off the Xanax, so his psychiatrist, whom I had great faith in, put him on a taper regimen for ten days. We now know this was extremely dangerous, that he could have died, and that he should have been weaned slowly over a course of at least a year.

But he did it in days, and the day after his last eighth of a pill, strange outward symptoms started to appear. Purposeless, repetitive movements as if he'd been set on fire. Weepiness. Pacing. Gruesome images and sounds in his mind and impulsive suicidal urges he'd never experienced before. Stroke like symptoms. The onset of tortuous nerve pain… and the beginning of a Kafkaesque journey towards a proper diagnosis.

Our first stop was a brilliant and compassionate physician and homeopath who gave Marcello a homeopathic remedy. It didn't touch the symptoms, so we went back to the original psychiatrist. She looked at him like… well, like he was crazy.

A month earlier, on the phone, she'd said, "Gee… this sounds like akathisia!" But when Marcello went back to her, rocking back and forth, begging for help, she said it wasn't possible to get akathisia from antidepressants. From antipsychotics, sure, but not from benign antidepressants. She thought whatever was wrong was "somatic" and suggested we get a second opinion. Meanwhile,

Fig. 2.1 (continued)

she prescribed a succession of meds designed to help with the strange movements, all of which made Marcello worse. (We now know that adding medications only exacerbates akathisia.)

We saw a second psychiatrist, who agreed this was likely somatic and suggested another antidepressant, which Marcello declined, understandably wary now of meds. He also suggested that Marcello would benefit from a month at his outpatient clinic where he'd receive various therapies, along with yoga and mindfulness, for forty thousand dollars.

My husband and I were up for it. But, in addition to being in constant pain, Marcello's sleep was becoming extremely erratic, and he absolutely couldn't see driving across L.A. twice a day in rush hour traffic to spend eight hours at the clinic. He'd always loved cars, loved driving, but his sensitivity to light and sound were increasing to the point where just being in a car was becoming impossible.

A third psychiatrist observed Marcello's movements and desperate state for five minutes, and immediately diagnosed akathisia. He regretfully informed us that the only "cure" was a high dosage of the potent antipsychotic Clozapine. He added that, though Marcello was not psychotic, he'd have to be hospitalized and closely monitored, as the drug could cause seizures, heart attack, lung clots, etc. But he assured us that the clinic where Marcello would be staying was so nice, he'd put his own daughter there.

The non-refundable fee would be a hundred thousand dollars. (One "side effect" of Clozapine he didn't mention, but which we later found on the net, is "a feeling of restlessness with an inability to sit still"... aka akathisia.)

By this time, Marcello was researching akathisia himself and becoming more frightened of medications. So, we moved on to a famous "integrative" psychiatrist and came home with a dozen supplements, prescribed via muscle testing. Marcello was told to take them all at once, which turned out to be a disaster. Unfortunately, this psychiatrist, whom he liked a lot, was busy moving houses and couldn't handle our many emails, so she suggested Marcello see a colleague who was "a genius at micro-dosing meds"—which, she assured us, would be safe.

The new psychiatrist was only seeing patients at a drug rehab where she was on staff. But since Marcello was experiencing "withdrawal" effects from the rapid Xanax taper, luckily, he was eligible for her rehab. We filled out the forms, packed him a bag, and headed across L.A. to the clinic, a run-down old Craftsman in a rough neighborhood.

It was staffed with alumni patients, recovering young drug addicts, and one of them gave us a tour. Marcello was kind of in shock and sat it out, but the young man's story of rehab really moved me. If only my son were a drug addict, and not allergic to medications, there'd be so much help out there! But the micro dosing psychiatrist was... well, she was a bitch. Never looked up from her computer, never looked at my son.

The house reeked of cigarettes and Clorox, and, since Marcello was developing strong chemical sensitivities now due to mast cell activation—a side effect of the akathisia—we just didn't have the heart to leave him there. So, we drove back home in rush hour traffic. Another two-hour assault on his injured central nervous system, which gave new meaning to the phrase, "Oh the traffic was hell."

Fig. 2.1 (continued)

After the drug rehab, we went to a peaceful holistic medical clinic just a few freeway exits away. They were calm and reassuring and gave him intravenous vitamins. We went to a renowned Israeli trauma therapist who diagnosed "trauma." We got to see the leading expert on "TMS" brain therapy who offered to zap his brain for a thousand dollars a go. Marcello saw a psychologist, via Facetime, who said he had "rage" and tried to get him to scream over Facetime. Another psychiatrist suggested CBT therapy. An Arab psychiatrist felt that joining his "community" would connect Marcello to his deeper self. And another psychiatrist suggested another med.

As he went from doctor to doctor, Marcello also got involved with a Facebook group called "Living with Akathisia" and a couple of other online groups like the "Benzodiazepine Information Coalition," "Neurotoxicity and Toxic Encephalopathy," and a group called "Cymbalta Hurts Worse."

Frankly, "Living with Akathisia" scared the hell out of me. People were making videos of their akathisia experience that looked like horror films. After much input from these groups and a great deal more research on his own about akathisia, he decided unequivocally that meds were not the way to go. After all, meds had proven toxic to him, causing akathisia in the first place.

His friends and ours were also weighing in, some offering their own diagnoses. The mother of the best friend with the cars had spoken to a couple of psychologist friends who'd never heard of akathisia, so she thought it was a "fake disease." Her son, who by now had ten cars and was traveling in a private jet, texted me that my son's blood was on my hands if I didn't commit him to a mental hospital.

One of the most promising doctors we encountered did indeed come through the friend of a friend of a friend. This doctor was an expert in a special kind of neurofeedback called Loreta. She practiced in a town an hour and a half from Los Angeles, but she assured us we were wasting money and hope if we were doing anything else, because Loreta was "the answer." She made a connection with Marcello, she listened, and had deep compassion. I was hopeful.

Because by this time, the outer manifestation of Marcello's torment was scaring us, and we were, indeed, considering hospitalization. My funny, wise, compassionate son was…gone. In his place was someone I couldn't reach, someone in an agony I could not fathom, someone filled with terror and, sometimes, rage.

The Loreta treatment was based on qEEG scans of Marcello's brain which showed "drastic abnormalities." The doctor was convinced she could help but would only work with him if he also saw a "brilliant integrative psychiatrist" with whom she worked as a team. And since this doctor practiced in another town, my husband and Marcello moved to a town in between the two doctors for three days a week.

Then the Loreta doctor went on a trip to Costa Rica, broke her back in the shower, and could not treat Marcello anymore. Like I said… Kafkaesque.

We did continue to see the integrative psychiatrist who was an expert on the brain and had no doubt that Marcello had akathisia caused by medication. Marcello bonded with him because he was young and open and was willing to prescribe supplements, slowly, one at a time, as opposed to meds.

Fig. 2.1 (continued)

At one point, the psychiatrist agreed with some folks on the Living with Akathisia site that a certain strain of marijuana might possibly help. After a few hits, it made Marcello run out into the rain in what *looked* like a true psychotic break—but was actually the akathisia being severely aggravated by the marijuana. Marcello recently told me that it was the most horrific night thus far, as he'd been filled with powerful urges to kill both his father and himself, and that he'd spent the night outside in the rain in an orchard to be safe.

This might be a good place to add that, before medication, he'd never gotten into a physical fight, never had a suicidal urge, and had always had a warm, close, and playful relationship with his father, who slept in his room now to keep watch, and loved him more than life itself.

Marcello was becoming sicker and sicker, developing severe reactions to foods, to supplements, to chemicals in the environment. Mosquito bites now caused anaphylaxis and sent him to the ER. But every ER we went to, and we went to several, said it was "anxiety." Each time, a kind doctor offered Ativan. Each time, we thanked them, declined, and left.

But one time was different. While my son and husband were waiting to check out of the ER, a psychiatric social worker who had examined Marcello, took them aside to another room. She said she could lose her job for telling them, but she also worked in a brain trauma center where she'd seen patients with akathisia who'd been put on a series of psych meds in hospitals… and, frankly, she'd seen their brains and bodies utterly destroyed. She quietly urged us to find another way.

Maybe the worst symptom of akathisia—for the parent, anyway—is "suicidal urges." And, finally, after months of incessant torture, and medical gaslighting, our son made an impulsive attempt. It was not a "serious attempt" according to the integrative psychiatrist, but it was serious enough for him to take over and call an ambulance.

Marcello spent ten days in the psych ward at UCLA. I remember looking back at him through a series of locked glass doors at the end of every visiting hour, seeing him grow smaller and smaller as we walked away. This was not like leaving my child at pre-school or summer camp. Akathisia had him. The State had him, legally. And I couldn't run back through the glass doors, pick him up in my arms, and whisk him away.

No two doctors could agree on a diagnosis. But they all wanted to give him meds. They didn't agree on which meds, but they were prepared to get a court order to administer… something. Interestingly, the nurses, who have the most interaction with patients, recognized his akathisia and told him they see it all the time.

When someone goes to the ER in severe physical pain, they are their own credible witness, and everyone believes them. But you're a whole lot less likely to be taken as a credible witness in a psych ward, especially if you have medication-induced akathisia, which can *look* like schizophrenia or psychosis.

Marcello recently told me that he was prepared to climb a barrier fence and jump off the hospital's twelve-story roof in the event that drugs were forced on him, as it would've exacerbated the akathisia to a point that would've been "far worse than death." And if he *were* to survive forced medication, he'd have to detox from the toxic drugs all over again, prolonging his recovery by years.

Fig. 2.1 (continued)

This was his thinking in the hospital, which I didn't know about at the time. Cause he was barely speaking to me. Cause I thought he should give the docs a chance.

His main doc at UCLA said, "his irrational fear of meds was a sign of severe OCD." And, to my eternal shame, I believed him over my son. Well, for a couple of days. After all, wouldn't OCD be better than akathisia—for which there is no treatment or cure?

We had a family meeting with the doctors, in which Marcello was not treated like credible witness by the experts. I remember he wouldn't look at me. This was particularly painful as we'd always been talkers. I'd always felt lucky to have a son who could go deep, who wasn't afraid of feelings, who said what he thought and felt, to his friends, his teachers, and, especially, to his parents.

He'd always been funny, irreverent, and could make people laugh despite themselves. Teachers were a bit baffled, but admired him. I heard more than once, always with a sigh, "I think we learned more from him than he could possibly have learned from us." And now we were *here* where no one believed him.

In retrospect, I think Marcello took that first pill to fit in. To tamp down the edges of a personality that felt more, saw more, questioned more, and spoke more truth. "More" than what was comfortable or convenient for others.

I remember his first psychiatrist calling me to run down the checklist for "bipolar" while he was sitting in there in her office. She just couldn't make him "fit" into a DSM diagnosis. She was the mother of a son my son's age, and I know she gave Marcello that first prescription because she wanted to ease his pain of trying to fit in.

When Marcello's insured days were up, UCLA suggested he go to the one private treatment center which would accept him without meds… and if that didn't work, he'd be sent back to UCLA where they'd get that court order to medicate.

He went to a private treatment center called Balance, near Malibu. I thought it was a lovely place. Good food, nice grounds, I was ready to check in for a nice rest myself. They "did not label him with a diagnosis," they were interested in him "as a whole person." With our insurance, we received a discounted offer for a thirty day stay at thirty thousand dollars.

All Marcello had to do was see their doctors and attend groups with other patients. But in the groups, he had to be still and attentive… which is impossible with akathisia. After five days of reactions to chemicals in the house, strict schedules he physically could not adhere to, and pressure to sit down and share like the other patients, (who were there for psychiatric disorders as opposed to neurological injuries), he ran.

Balance reported him "missing" to the police. He called to let us know he was "safe." He'd fled to a hotel an hour away, and we raced over. We spoke to the people at Balance on the phone, and they advised us to let the police come to the hotel and take back him to UCLA. Marcello overheard enough to know the police were on the way, and he ran again. Shot right by me with the yellow backpack he got in Copenhagen on that trip of a lifetime.

Fig. 2.1   (continued)

I started screaming. The hotel maids tried to comfort me. My husband and I looked everywhere, but he was gone. Then the police came.

My husband and I had a decision to make. Help them find our son and cuff him and take him in a police car to UCLA to be force-medicated... or let our son determine his own fate. There had been a lot of moments over the past months that forced us to ask ourselves, "Who are you going to trust?" "Whose counsel can you rely on?" "Who do you believe, the doctor or your son?" This moment was the hardest.

Our son was now twenty-two. Nothing, nothing we had tried had worked to alleviate his suffering, certainly no med. We went home and prayed. By this time, we believed in nothing. But you pray anyway.

Oh, this is as good a time as any to mention we had received an eviction notice from our landlady because of all the noise in our house, and the ambulance and all, but I digress.

Marcello called from the airport and said he was about to board a plane to Oregon, where he'd spent much of his childhood. But that night he showed up at our house in L.A. As I mentioned, one of the main features of akathisia is extreme sensitivity to stimulation of any kind, so he could barely make it through airport security.

Still, the next morning, I went downstairs to his room and he was gone. We got a call from Oregon, where he hoped to find refuge until he could help us understand what he knew, and what he was learning from other long-term sufferers, about akathisia. There'd be no more running, no more threat of forced drugging. And, in hindsight, his father and I know this was the wisest decision he could have made.

At the time, however, Balance suggested we call a woman in the Midwest who could organize an "intervention" in Oregon and get him back to UCLA. We declined. Our son wasn't crazy. His brain and central nervous system were not as well as they were before Cymbalta and Prozac and Xanax... But he wasn't delusional, and he'd managed not to hurt anyone or himself, even when gaslighted by doctors and restrained, which was a miracle.

By now, he'd studied akathisia more deeply than the doctors who'd been treating him. And beyond all that... He was a human being. It seemed to me that to force anyone to take medication, (that the FDA classifies as dangerous), against their will, robs them of dominion over their own body and mind. What more basic right does a human being have? I couldn't call the woman in the Midwest.

Since January 2020, Marcello has been in Oregon. He started seeing his old family doctor, who, ironically, has had two family members survive akathisia and thought he could help. When he first got to Oregon, Marcello was able to do more things for himself living in the center of a small town. The disabling akathisia was the same, but he felt safer, part of a familiar place.

Karen came to live with him. He started HBOT, (hyperbaric oxygen therapy), which didn't help but didn't hurt either. He could even meet a friend for a short walk near the Airbnb where he was staying. Then Covid hit.

Fig. 2.1 (continued)

Ironically, I was the original screenwriter of "Girl, Interrupted," and as I write this, I realize it's "Boy, Interrupted" for sure. A young man's life is interrupted by some pills that promised to make life better. That's what *happened*.

But the writer in me is always looking for some... meaning. If I can just wrest some goddamn meaning from what's happening, I can deal. So when I look at what happened to Marcello, I think about what we are doing to ourselves as a culture—as we wrestle with the lure of the American Dream. The pills we need to keep chasing it. The greed on the part of the drug companies that fuels our discontent and encourages our striving.

And then, in contrast to the American Dream... there's the pull of the natural world. It's fascinating to me that Marcello's two best friends happened to embody these two different pulls. And maybe it's no accident that he started this chapter of his life in New York City, where you have to take a train to the planetarium, and has wound up in small town Oregon where you can just look up and see stars.

Akathisia is an incredibly complex neurological injury. But, according to experts in the field of neuroplasticity, such as psychiatrist Norman Doidge, author of *The Brain That Changes Itself*, the brain is really miraculous. If you remove the neurotoxicity—from the meds, from our processed food, from the chemicals in our environment—even a badly damaged brain can regenerate.

If you then give the brain what it *needs*—real food, pure water, clean air, low stress—it can heal. And aren't these the things that all humans need? Not to mention the poor planet? Might this be some bit of meaning we can wrest from the pandemic?

Marcello and I are telling this story in the interest of furthering "informed consent." Because if this could happen to him, it could happen to anyone. At this time, the only conventional "treatment" for akathisia is more medications which cause akathisia. Sufferers talk of being "polydrugged"—given one drug to offset the negative effects of another—and they liken it to using gasoline to put out a fire.

They are not being cured, and, because the condition is so terrifying to others, many sufferers lose their families and friends. This loss drives many to suicide. And again, these are mostly people with no history of attempted suicide before taking medication. They don't want to *die*, they just want the anguish of akathisia to end. But what about people who *do* have mental illness and develop akathisia *on top of that*? What about people of color, or poor people, who don't have access to information and support—what the hell kind of shot do *they* have?

Here's what haunts me: Could hundreds of thousands of suicides have been prevented if people had had "informed consent" before starting meds?

What might informed consent entail? There is a major Australian study by Dr. Yolande Lucire and Christopher Crotty entitled "Antidepressant-induced akathisia related homicides associated with diminishing mutations in metabolizing genes of the CYP450 family." (Whew.) Based on over a hundred and twenty subjects, the study shows links between both suicides and homicides in akathisia patients who have the CYP450 gene variation.

The authors state that "prescribing antidepressants without knowing about CYP450 genotypes is like giving blood transfusions without matching for ABO groups." They conclude that it's essential

Fig. 2.1   (continued)

to look into a patient's genetics before prescribing. So. What if our son had had the proper tests, and someone with the training to interpret them, *before* being handed his prescription?

The Australian study notes that drug companies actually reject people with the CYP450 variation from their trials. They know that for these people the drug will be toxic, and they don't want these folks to "contaminate" (lower) the success rates in their studies. They do not, however, warn the public about the dangers associated with this gene variation when the drug is marketed. (Yes, this is actually allowed.)

According to the Australian study, psychiatric drugs are "prescribed by clinicians educated by drug company representatives and key opinion leaders who receive substantial benefits from the makers of these drugs." So, in order for the patient to be fully informed, the psychiatrist has to be fully informed… And does a multi-billion-dollar drug industry really want that?

Ultimately, the best way to treat akathisia is to prevent it from ever happening. And we know the pharmaceutical industry does not want *that*.

On August 19, 2021, Marcello will be two years off of any medication, after having been on meds for a total of three and a half months. He can't drive, can't focus on a movie or TV, can't listen to music or read a book, can't tolerate the foods he used to whip up into incredible meals, can't hike or climb mountains.

His sleep has been disrupted by a potentially permanent circadian rhythm disorder called "non-24," which basically means it spins around the clock, an hour or two later every day, *if* he is able to sleep at all. Every hour he's awake is devoted to surviving the moment-to-moment torment of akathisia.

Karen, the friend he grew up hiking and camping with, was with him for seven months. When she left for a job in San Diego, his dad and I moved to Oregon, as he can't live alone. He needs to apply for disability, but, with the disaster wrought by Covid on millions, his chances are slim.

And if *he* were to contract Covid? It's not likely his system could handle it. His doctor doesn't think he could handle the vaccine either. Which is why, despite everything we don't know about the long-term impact of the vaccines, and everything I've learned about Big Pharma, you bet I'm going for that shot… to keep him safe.

When Marcello describes akathisia, he says one of the most insidious effects is that it has completely hijacked his ability to feel anything good, anything human. Yes, he can see the stars in Oregon, only now they overwhelm and agitate him, a cruel reminder of something that used to evoke wonder. Same with people. He knows he loves us, loves Karen, he just can't *feel* it.

So, no, I can't talk about a "happy ending." Not yet. We hold fast to the research that says that in time the brain does heal. If I can't slay the goddess Akathisia, I'll just have to outwait her.

Meanwhile… Marcello has managed to write and produce a PSA for The Akathisia Alliance which you can watch right here. He's a whistle blower in the making, speaking about akathisia on social media and to anyone who'll listen. He's not just passionate about getting this information out there, it's what he lives for.

Fig. 2.1 (continued)

1. How would you include the information in the article in a formulation?
2. Which parts of the information contained in the article stand out for you and why?
3. Which issues raised in the article make you want to find out more information and how would you do this if you were working with the service user or their family?

Student responses to these questions are summarised and presented in Table 2.2.

Reflections on This Exercise

Students have explored the accounts of Marcello's mother and Marcello's experiences. Questions around choice, information and trying to gain understanding around events and experiences have been highlighted, as well as power imbalances. These outlooks are helpful in formulation processes. Students who participated in this exercise found this a very thought-provoking experience which supported them in researching the issues raised in further detail, reflecting on their aims as registered practitioners.

Chapter Summary

This chapter examined the literature on the use of formulation in mental health nursing and services and teams in which mental health nurses practise. In addition, some approaches and models of formulation have been outlined. An exercise on mental health nursing students outlooks and preferences for models of formulation has been presented as well as exploring student views on a mother's description of the difficulties and distress of her son experiencing Akathisia. This has given an opportunity for reflection to identify areas requiring further inquiry and to try and make sense of reported experiences. We hope this has also given you an opportunity to reflect on your own views, values and outlooks in relation to the content presented here.

Key Points for Reflection
1. Have you read any more recent research or articles which report on contemporary use of using formulation both in the MDT and by mental health nurses?
2. Do you have any preferences for formulation models, if so why is this?
3. What were your responses to the article by Lisa Loomer?
4. Is there anything you will take away from this chapter and apply to your own practice or outlooks?

Table 2.2 Mental health nursing student responses to the article by Loomer (2021)

Question	A sample of student comments	Analysis and summary of responses
1. How would you include this information (from the article) in a formulation?	"Marcello had done a lot of research himself. He'd been in discussion groups and had a great understanding of what akathisia is. Understanding his history within the health sector and knowing that he was a much greater expert on akathisia than myself, I would form a formulation by asking him where he would like to go at this point. From online discussion boards, it's likely he would have access to people who have tried various successful and unsuccessful therapies to therefore have an opinion on how he would like to move forward, and what interventions he's willing to try." "There is a lot of information in this article about what Marcello has tried, and what has not worked for him. It would be important to include all the things that have made it worse for Marcello and what have had no effect—in the formulation. I would also ask Marcello what he thinks, as he knows more than doctors. He knows how he is feeling and also knows what he doesn't want to try. It is also apparent that there are some things he may not be able to handle because of the akathisia and he is the best person to tell us that." "I would speak to both parents and Marcello together and separately to gain more insight into their struggle with Akathisia. With there being an extensive history of medications and interventions, which have been used with and without asking Marcello his opinions surrounding them, I would discuss what he would think would work best for him. It would be doubtful Marcello would accept or be trusting of medications straight away so I doubt this would be an initial option. As he is involved with social media platforms specifically for Akathisia, it would be beneficial to know how these have helped Marcello come to terms with Akathisia and if group therapy would be an option, particularly if there are groups specifically designed for this diagnosis. Also, to speak with the parents alone as financially any treatment would be at a hefty cost, and from the history of treatments already given they may be in extensive debt which could have an impact on any future treatment." "I would use all of the information in the article as the viewpoint of his mother, I would however want to hear his story, I would encourage him to share some history as I feel that the information we have is recent and post medication. We don't have much information of what was going on for him prior to medication."	Students identified the following as important for inclusion in a formulation: • Asking the person about what is important to them and putting them at the centre of the discussion. • Giving space and time to talk to Marcello and his parents together and alone. • Explore further Marcello's experiences before he started taking medication.

(continued)

Table 2.2 (continued)

Question	A sample of student comments	Analysis and summary of responses
2. Which parts of the information contained in the article stand out for you and why?	"What stood out to me most seemed to be that Marcello wasn't being listened to. He had the knowledge of akathisia and the understanding that treatment would become difficult with the use of medication being ruled out and talking therapies being hard for him to be able to participate in, yet the professionals he saw believed they knew best and continued to try to put Marcello in these situations anyway. It was particularly difficult to read about Marcello almost being forced medication treatment if the alternative therapies were unsuccessful. There appeared to be such a heavy reliance on the fact that medication would help him if they could just find the right one, instead of listening to Marcello and accepting that this might not be the case." "I was shocked at the amount of medication Marcello had been prescribed, and how many times these had been changed, along with how quickly he was took off them and straight onto something new. It has not given his body time to be weaned of the current medication before his body had to absorb something new. The fact that Marcello, despite doing his own research and from reading the article he seemed to have done quite a lot into Akathisia—his voice was not heard, he was dismissed and mis diagnosed as somatic. The prices for some of the treatment as well, some being thousands of pounds was shocking within itself." "The amount of missed diagnoses and various medications given to Marcello from numerous professionals who were not willing to listen to him as a person and instead only see him as a list of symptoms. Also, the amount of money, which was charged for Marcello's treatment, and how much money pharmaceutical industries make on psychiatric medication—could be one of the reasons why they are prescribed so easily when there is so much money to be made."	Students identified these prominent issues including; • The power imbalance between the professionals and Marcello. • That professionals did not listen to Marcello. • The ethical issues of the prescribed medications and financial implications.

| 3. Which issues raised in the article make you want to find out more information and how would you do this if you were working with the service user or their family? | "After reading the article, I'd like to know what has helped other people be able to live with their akathisia, and whether or not time is the only way for them to return to some sense of normalcy. I'm interested in finding if there is a therapy that can help akathisia. In order to find out this information in practice, I'd talk to the service user and their family as they're likely to be the experts in the subject and try to understand it from their point of view, I'd then research further to see what I can bring to their care as well."

"I would like to know how other people have developed akathisia as it sounds like it can be the results of a lot of different medications. It would also be good to know if anything has worked for them to relieve the symptoms. The mention of a specific gene is also interesting."

"Why he needed antidepressants to begin with and was any other therapies introduced or suggested before the doctor went to medication, was the doctor a general practitioner or psychiatric doctor, was there support offered or groups, seems many other pathways could have been explored before medications."

"I want to increase my knowledge on medications, I feel that medication should be monitored more closely and I was surprised to read about the implications of genetics."

"It was difficult to read and know that institutions can be so poorly prepared to help someone who has the knowledge of how he's suffering, yet ignore what he's saying and attempt to put him in further pain believing they know best. In terms of the medication being tried in this article, I've been considering becoming a nursing prescriber for a while now, and reading this is making me re-evaluate my decision. It has made me recognise that prescribing should be done very carefully and has made me understand the saying 'the first rule of prescribing is to try not to prescribe'. I'm going to take on board this article when I make the decision further into my career as to whether this is an area of nursing I'd like to participate in."

"This article shows how dangerous medication can be and also is a reminder that a diagnosis and then the prescription of a medication is often given too quickly. It also shows how people can often focus too much on putting people in a box instead of listening to them and thinking about all the possible explanations for how they are feeling." | Students identified that they would like to learn more about Akathisia and how it is managed or cured. Students questioned what initial support was offered to Marcello before medication was prescribed.

Reflections on personal motivations, outlooks and values in supporting people were discussed. |

References

Barker, P. (2001). The Tidal Model: The lived experience in person-centred mental health nursing care. *Nursing Philosophy, 2*(3), 213–223.

British Psychological Society. (2010). *Clinical psychology leadership development framework*. British Psychological Society.

Clark, L., & Clarke, T. (2014). Realizing nursing: A multimodal biopsychpharmacosocial approach to psychiatric nursing. *Journal of Psychiatric and Mental Health Nursing, 21*, 564–571.

Cox, L. (2020). Use of individual formulation in mental health practice. *Mental Health Practice.* https://doi.org/10.7748/mhp.2020.e1515

Crowe, M., Carlyle, D., & Farmer, R. (2008). Clinical formulation for mental health nursing practice. *Journal of Psychiatric and Mental Health Nursing, 15*, 800–807.

Harris, H., & Barraclough, B. (1998). Excess mortality in mental disorder. *The British Journal of Psychiatry, 173*, 11–53.

Hartley, S. (2021). Using team formulation in mental health practice. *Mental Health Practice.* https://doi.org/10.7748/mhp.2021.e1516

Jones, S., Howard, L., & Thornicroft, G. (2008). Diagnostic overshadowing: Worse physical health care for people with mental illness. *Acta Psychiatrica Scandinavica, 118*, 169–171.

Loomer, L. (2021). Boy, interrupted: A story of Akathisia. *Mad in America.* https://www.madinamerica.com/2021/06/boy-interrupted-a-story-of-akathisia/

McTiernan, K., Jackman, L., Robinson, L., & Thomas, M. (2021). A thematic analysis of the multidisciplinary team understanding of the 5P Team Formulation Model and its evaluation on a psychosis rehabilitation unit. *Community Mental Health Journal, 57*, 579–588.

Peplau, H. (1952). *Interpersonal relations in nursing*. Putnam.

Williams, C., & Chellingsworth, M. (2010). *CBT: A clinician's guide to using the five areas approach*. Hodder Arnold.

Yeandle, J., Fawkes, L., Beeby, R., Gordon, C., & Challis, E. (2015). A collaborative formulation framework for service users with personality disorders. *Mental Health Practice, 18*, 25–28.

Three Functions of Using Psychoanalytic and Systemically Informed Perspectives in Case Formulation: Ways of Thinking About Distress in Others, Our Own Reflexive Contribution and Collaborative Formulation

Claire Barber

Key Learning Points
- Formulation as an ideological structure
- Steps in the process of formulation
- Domains of thinking—a floorplan of the relationships between theoretical spaces in the process of formulation
- Prioritising contextual factors including the 5Ps and risk
- Choosing the most helpful quadrant to focus upon
- Reflexivity and collaboration
- A family genogram and making sense of Chloe's story
- Trauma Informed Approach and Adverse Childhood Experiences
- Medical, Social, Cognitive Behavioural and Psychoanalytic and Systemically informed Domains—assessment and interventions
- Listening to the story in relation to risk assessment of suicidality and self-harm
- Communication patterns, The Social GGRRAAACCEEESSS and LUUUTT models
- Formulation as a mitigating process for burnout and directionless practice
- Formulation as a tool for group supervision / case discussion

C. Barber (✉)
City, University of London, London, UK
e-mail: Claire.Barber@city.ac.uk

© The Author(s), under exclusive license to Springer Nature Switzerland AG 2024
V. Howard, L. Alfred (eds.), *Formulation in Mental Health Nursing*,
https://doi.org/10.1007/978-3-031-59956-9_3

Introduction

This chapter will consider *some* psychological, psychoanalytical and psychodynamic perspectives of formulation. The words are essentially interchangeable depending upon your theoretical frame of reference. In this chapter the focus is upon theories of identity and emotional development; systemic and relational influences; and the act of *doing* formulation as a reflexive group process. Formulation is a framework to invite evidence-based hypothesis and thinking that can challenge assumptions and invite new ideas and knowledge and focus our conversations, assessments and interventions. The utility of group formulation and discussion affords our thinking and about the person's experience of distress. The chapter asserts that one perspective is not enough to understand the whole story. The focus is on developing knowledge and use of case formulation as a means of collaboratively understanding a person's experience of mental and or physical distress and illness, whether in crisis or longer-term situations: from cognitive behavioural, medical, psychological and social perspectives. Some authors may differ in the way they name the different domains of formulation as CBT, Psychodynamic, Systemic and Integrative (Johnson & Dallos, 2014) and as a consequence favour different influences; but the process, i.e. *the act of doing* formulation is what is foregrounded; the process of exploration is the same regardless of your theoretical or professional position. I have used this approach in my own clinical practice, in the teaching of undergraduate and postgraduate students and continued professional development of clinicians in practice to frame discussions in group supervision for many years. I never fail to be impressed and captivated by the level of critical thinking and compassionate willingness of students and clinicians to be self-effacing about the theoretical models we feel wedded to, and a readiness to consider assumptions we all hold about personhood, illness and expected outcomes. This chapter may be of use to new and experienced clinicians. It may not offer new theoretical knowledge to experienced clinicians but prompt each to consider ways of working—using formulation as a structure to think together, assess and work with individuals and families referred with mental and physical health difficulties. I have been inspired by, and learnt from, those with whom I have had the privilege to work with: colleagues, students and people with lived and living experience. I could not have done my job without involving the thinking of others. There is a case example of a family's story which is shared to illustrate the ideas offered in this chapter.

Formulation as an Ideological Structure

Formulation is an ideological structure that can provide clinicians with the flexibility to consider multiple factors and theoretical frameworks and can be used in conjunction with other assessment tools, strategies and diagnostic criteria in assessment of physical and mental illness. It is an attempt to deconstruct and reconstruct what might be the person's experience and inform further assessment and intervention. A criticism of this approach is that it might be a reductive account of a person's life, nevertheless, we meet people who are ill or in distress, regardless of which 'door' of health or social care through which people come to our attention. Our professional mandate and moral obligation is to consider opportunities for recovery and support. Formulation can assist us to 'map' what has happened, how we might help the person, their families or carers, and how our current assessment and intervention can influence future health outcomes.

One definition of the term formulation is *"the action of creating or preparing something"* (Oxford English Dictionary, 2023). It is a creative inclusive process, not a unidirectional conclusion from the clinician's expert position. A singular linear approach to formulation does not consider the service user's voice, their lived and living experience, understanding and expertise; nor does it consider the perspectives of other colleagues. Another definition says formulation is *"a mixture prepared according to a formula"* (Oxford English Dictionary, 2023) in this respect the process of formulation helps us to consider the importance of different ingredients (multiple hypothesis—held lightly) that form multidimensional possibilities of understanding and working.

The First Step of Formulation

This involves deconstructing all aspects: signs, symptoms, conversations of the person's difficulty and considers ideas that each lens, theoretical paradigm affords. We should question which of the different domains we tend to favour and sometimes recalibrate our formulation, mindful of our own professional or theoretical bias, inviting ideas and open our thinking to other perspectives. The task of formulation is to reconstruct the salient parts of the *'mixture'* in an attempt to co-create a cohesive understanding relationship between practitioners, the service user, the theory and the service resources available to us. However, the task can feel overwhelming. The complexity of a person's life story and why they are now in need of help may lead us to grasp at the first likely explanation of a situation; an answer which may not ultimately be in service of the person but meets our own needs or the productivity of the service rather than quality of care. We need to remember that although formulation is a helpful approach; it is not a magic 8 ball that once shaken will produce an answer. Nonetheless, using formulation in assessment and evaluation can prompt us to consider the foundations and each brick of our thinking about the person's difficulty, illness and distress. The significance of each part and how they influence or intersect is the process of formulation. The job of the clinician is to be open to feedback, invite reflective and reflexive thinking and be agile between the different domains.

Formulation has an influential role in maintaining wellbeing for the promotion and prevention of future mental distress, therefore, due consideration of protective factors and risk factors associated with poor mental health is required. It is crucial that we hold all factors in mind when choosing to focus more specifically upon one. Contextual and environmental thinking can be of equal relevance in our deliberations; and may prove to be the areas we need to divert our attention to in our ongoing assessment and evaluation.

DOMAINS OF THINKING

The theoretical and contextual factors in Fig. 3.1 are suggestions and should be collaboratively co-produced and revised. The map can be used as an aide-memoire for discussion and group supervision.

Once we have 'mapped' known contextual factors about the person, their family and relationships, due consideration must be given to prioritising information relevant to the '5P's' (Peters, 2020), i.e. presenting problems, predisposing, precipitating, perpetuating and protective factors that holds equal primacy in our work. Each domain of formulation must include evaluation of risk of self-harm, suicidality and safeguarding. Thinking about risk and our reflexive bias are integral parts of all assessment and formulation processes.

The National Institute of Health and Care Excellence (NICE) (2022) guidelines about self-harm cover "assessment, management and preventing recurrence for children, young people and adults and includes those with mental health problems, neurodevelopment disorder or learning disability". The Royal College of Psychiatry (RCP) (2023) warned against 'fundamentally flawed' categorical tick box declaration of 'low risk' or 'no risk' of suicide;

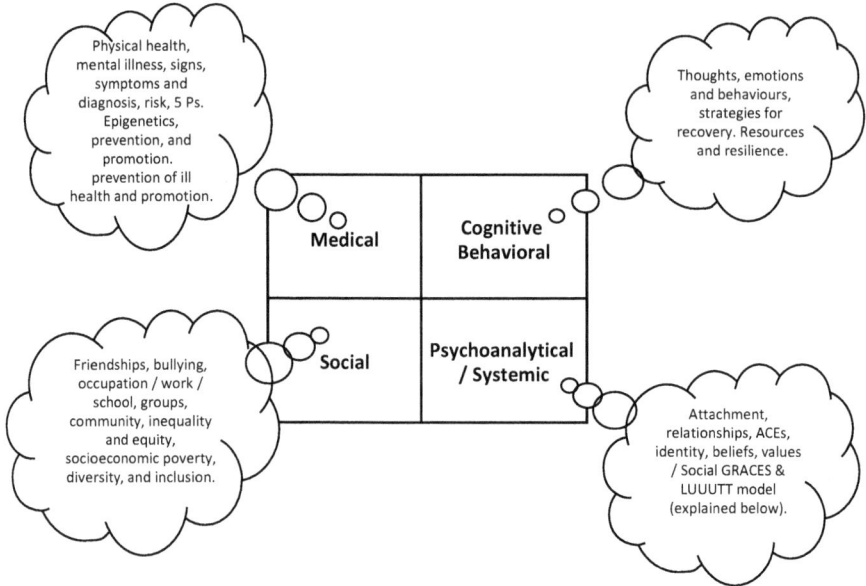

Fig. 3.1 A floorplan of the relationships between theoretical spaces in the process of formulation

which carries the possibility of missing life-saving support. We must therefore question practices inherent in our own training, beliefs, professional, lived experiences and a tendency to foreground some theories above others, if we are to become more co-productive and expansive in our deliberations about care.

It is professionally and morally incumbent upon us to constantly challenge our own thinking, and invite discourse from others, in service of the people with whom we work. We need to be cognisant of all aspects of the person's distress and illness across the life course, even when this is at a speculative or hypothetical stage of formulation. Consideration of past and present relationships and environmental factors needs to inform our assessment. Appreciation of epigenetics, an area of research which is now beginning to permeate contemporary practice formulation, takes into account how environmental experiences influence affect how much or how little of the chemical markers in our DNA are expressed in our genes. The nature versus nurture debate is no longer relevant in an 'either or' sense, it is both, and offers explanation about why genetically identical twins can display different behaviours, cognitive ability, skills, achievements and health attributes. Attachment experiences and environments in which a child develops can reconfigure gene expression from both positive and negative experiences, leaving unique epigenetic 'signatures' which can be temporary or permanent. Restorative relationships and lifestyle changes can significantly increase emotional and biological resilience and activate genetic potential (Jawaid et al., 2018; National Scientific Council, 2010). Knowing this can engender hopeful, productive approaches to formulation and practice.

The process of formulation informs future questions and assessment when underpinned by theory and research. However, we must strive to be open-minded enough not to rule factors in or out in a binary fashion based upon *our* clinical traditions, including the way we clinically label our involvement. Formulation invites us to consider what *might be* the person's presentation in relation to *their* past experiences, including their experiences of services. The *way* we meet with people is more important than *where* we meet people. Recommendations from the RCP (2020, p. 3) "Side by Side: A UK-wide consensus statement on working together to help patients with mental health needs in acute hospitals" urge: "*All healthcare professionals must work together to eradicate terms such as 'medically fit' or 'medical clearance'. The terms 'fit for assessment', 'fit for review' or 'fit for discharge' should be used instead to ensure parallel working*". They warn that this use of shorthand only refers to the person having no medical needs and does not mitigate against possible diagnostic overshadowing and risks giving false assurance. The "Treat as One" (2017) guidance refers to timely assistance for people with existing conditions and the needs for collaborative working across different disciplines.

Practical use of formulation can assist our appreciation of the experiences of individuals who are struggling with their emotional, mental, physical, and social identity and health care needs. Formulation enables clinicians to be both independent reflexive learners and teachers, lending their professional knowledge to exercise initiative and professional responsibility in collaborative decision making. The process enables us to appraise the utility of case formulation within the context of mental health services, apply aetiology of common mental health disorders, legislation, guidelines and research. It invites us to examine how the different theoretical perspectives of case formulation contribute to compassionate, culturally sensitive ways of working that inform interventions and appreciate the uniqueness of physical and psychological distress.

The act of formulation can imply the clinician's assertion of expert knowledge—the power to determine what is right, what is important and what is not. Just as supervision does not mean we have *super*-vision but the privilege to listen and to think together in a way that people we care for can feel metaphorically held, listened to and thought about. The image below shows how each quadrant increases or decreases when we populate the aperture or field of vision in each domain. What we do not know is sometimes as important to record as what is known (Fig. 3.2).

When favouring a Psychoanalytic and Systemic informed view, ideas from Bowlby's "Attachment theory" (Bowlby, 1988) and Erikson's "Eight stages of psychosocial developmental" (1964) were helpful to consider in relation to the case example given below. Systemic Psychotherapy and Family Therapy concepts were also considered in relation to trauma informed and emotionally focused practice of formulation.

These ideas are relatable in four contextual ways:

1. about the person, carers and families we work with;
2. about ourselves (clinicians) and how we might be experienced by others;
3. about the organisations in which we work; and
4. about the wider contextual societal discourses that may be germane to our understanding.

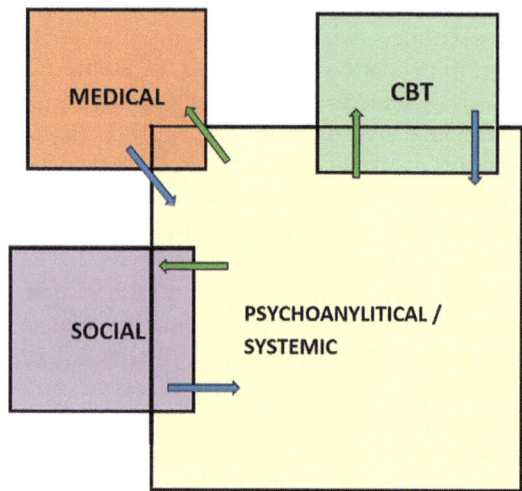

Fig. 3.2 Choosing the most helpful quadrant to focus upon

These four aspects can be useful theoretical positions to reflect upon and enable a more emotionally focused perception of trauma and the living experience of mental and physical illness and distress. The implications for practice, the culture of learning and thinking together should be flexibly applied to complement, not replace, action when there is a need to intervene and respond to emergency in either medical or safeguarding crisis.

Often the stories we hear in our work are drenched in sorrow and distress. We can become overwhelmed by the sheer volume of different discourses to the point that it can be challenging to hold hope. Nonetheless, these ideas not only bring colour and depth to our thinking but compassion and emotionally focused practice. To visualise an alternate way of thinking about the process of formulation is to imagine a stained-glass window. The work of artists like **Marc Chagall created stained-glass windows in the incredible St. Stephan Church, Mainz Germany 1978–1985** (images in Forestier et al., 2016); the historical and cultural significance of which are immense. They illuminate the renewal of friendship between France and Germany after the Second World War and the importance of reconciliation and harmony. As a Jewish artist, Chagall's message *"transcends religious themes to heal, and radiate a spirit of friendship, optimism, hope and joy of life"* is humbling as *"colours speak directly to our way of life, because they tell of optimism, hope, joy of life"* (Father Klaus Mayer, 1978–1975 Priest at St. Stephen's Church). To use this image as a metaphor for the framework of formulation—without the lead, however beautifully each pane of glass has been painted, the overall image and meaning are not contained. Without the glass there is only a black frame. Each part is fragile but strengthened and held by the framework. It is crucial that we respectfully hold lightly each part, idea, and contribution to the whole story and listen to the telling. The third dimension of this creative process is provided by the service user's illumination so that the true depth of colour may be genuinely understood and appreciated. The structure of the formulation process can give direction and substance to that hope.

REFLEXIVITY AND COLLABORATION

Formulation offers an opportunity to become more self-aware and ultimately effective in meeting the needs of the people we work with and for. The use of reflexivity is explained by Kadushin (1992, 2002) and requires us to consider our own bias and privilege, i.e. what we see in someone, or something may say more about us than the person or thing we are observing. Noticing what is evoked in us can be helpful data, e.g. when this forms part of the formulation discussion it can help us to explore and value difference, concerns for social justice, and alternate lenses through which to hypothesise and formulate without rigidity. Critical thinking within collaborative formulation mirrors the feedback process in group supervision. It is a structure for effective case discussion and a commitment to a learning-centred ethical practice and professional development. Reflexivity requires us to consciously examine our own subjective point of view, failure to do so could impact the outcome.

Formulation is an act of exploration and collaboration of meaning-making or co-production, that invites the voice of the service user's lived experience and that of other colleagues informed by theory and practice experience. Through the action of mapping our thinking, we can reach a point of deeper understanding and responsive feedback. Moving the boarders and increasing the aperture of our overall understanding of the act of formulation is reliant upon feedback from others. Assessing the *facts* through discussion is a part of the collaborative nature of formulation. However, we need to start conversations from a position of compassionate questioning about aspects of people's lives that may have been reported in the past as *truths* and populate the different domains with new and *known* descriptors. The destigmatising aspect of the process should emphasise capabilities and consider where people have been failed to be cared for across their lifespan, resulting in self-stigma which can hamper an individual's belief in recovery. As with many approaches to assessment, its original vogue and intention needs reviving to encompass reflexivity from the clinician, the service, political, environmental and socially constructed influences upon understanding of human experience.

Formulation can help us to adopt a **Trauma Informed Approach** (Clark et al., 2015; Oral et al., 2010). The principles of a trauma informed practice are: *safety; trustworthiness and transparency; collaboration and mutuality; empowerment and having a voice and choice.* **Adverse Childhood Experiences** (ACEs) can result in short- and/or long-term negative physical and mental illness and poorer health outcomes into adulthood. Research over the past forty years into ACEs focuses upon the ten most common experiences in childhood that include: child abuse (emotional neglect, physical and sexual abuse), household dysfunction (interpersonal domestic violence, substance abuse, parental mental illness, criminality, or parental absence), extreme poverty, bullying, school and community violence, traumatic loss of a loved one, sudden and frequent relocation, serious accidents, life threatening childhood illness/injury, pornography (exposure or participation), natural disaster, kidnapping, war, refugee camps and terrorism (Tully et al., 2021; Dube et al., 2001; Kessler et al., 2010; Oral et al., 2010). Consideration of the impact that ACEs have upon people can help us to begin to understand trauma, reduce myopic explanations of presenting physical and mental illness and distress, accommodate complexity in our thinking and engender trauma-informed, emotionally focused formulation and practice.

The case example given in this chapter is not fictional but anonymised sufficiently for the family to have given their consent and pseudonyms have been used. Specific clinical details are therefore not elaborated upon but referred to in a broad sense to articulate the process of formulation and application of theory. The story provides a psychoanalytic understanding of the person using Bowlby's Attachment theory, Erikson's theory of personality/emotional development and risk-taking behaviour were assessed in terms of depression, social anxiety, self-harm and current safeguarding.

CHLOE'S STORY

Chloe is a 13-year-old girl who was referred to CAMHS for an assessment of self-harm and suicidality, following an overdose. She was subsequently diagnosed with Depression and Social Anxiety Disorder (ICD-11) (International Classification of Diseases 2019/2021). The transgenerational mental health problems that existed within the family, include historical sexual abuse and ACEs experienced by her mother (although not known to Chloe or others in the family at the time of referral). These were later understood to have impacted upon Chole's presenting mental health difficulties and the family's story. Chloe's mother and Chloe's uncles experienced sexual abuse from their father as children. This was never spoken about at the time. Carol, Chloe's mother, left the family home when both her parents died at 17-years-old. She has had no contact with her older brothers or any other family members since she left. Carol and Tom, Chloe's father, met when Carol was 19 and they had two daughters, Emma and Chloe. Although divorced after 8 years they remain friends. Carol met Mark, her second husband, when Chloe was 5 and Emma was 11 years old (Fig. 3.3).

Initial formulation (using Fig. 3.1) charted the following concerns in each domain:

MEDICAL domain: Chloe had clear symptoms of Depression (DSM-5, F32) (American Psychiatric Association, 2013); depressed mood and loss of interest or pleasure (in friendships and activities); hypersomnia; fatigue, feelings of worthlessness, lack of concentration (at school and home) and Non-Suicidal Self-Injury (NSSI) (in the form of cuts to her forearms and overdose without thought of suicide but a wish to be taken care of). Social Anxiety Disorder (ICD-11) was also diagnosed; her primary symptoms included increased heart rate in social situations (school) as described by Chloe but not present on examination; hyperventilation and nausea (Chloe had a fear of being sick in public) in social situations where she felt she was being observed. Chloe's symptoms caused clinically significant distress for her and her family, resulting in impairment in personal, family, social and educational functioning and worrying about the future. Chloe was at a developmental age of transition from childhood to adolescence. It is helpful to consider Chloe's capacity for emotional regulation and risk taking behaviour in neurodevelopmental terms, i.e. in conjunction with dopamine theory and social versus physical risk. Emotional regulation is influenced by healthy levels of stress, acclimatising the infant/child to biologically manage stress; however sustained low levels of stimuli are as damaging as persistently high levels of stress. It is important to be reminded that synaptic/axonal pruning naturally takes place in the adolescent developing brain (Sisk & Romeo, 2019; Siegel, 2020). 'Responding to Childhood Trauma' (The Lancet Psychiatry, 2022) points us towards Herman's work on trauma and recovery and informed Complex PTSD (ICD-11).

MEDICAL assessment and intervention: Chloe was initially prescribed a short course of anti-depressants and she was referred to CAMHS following an NSSI overdose of paracetamol. On World Suicide Prevention Day (2023) the RCP called upon all mental health services to ensure that all patients with

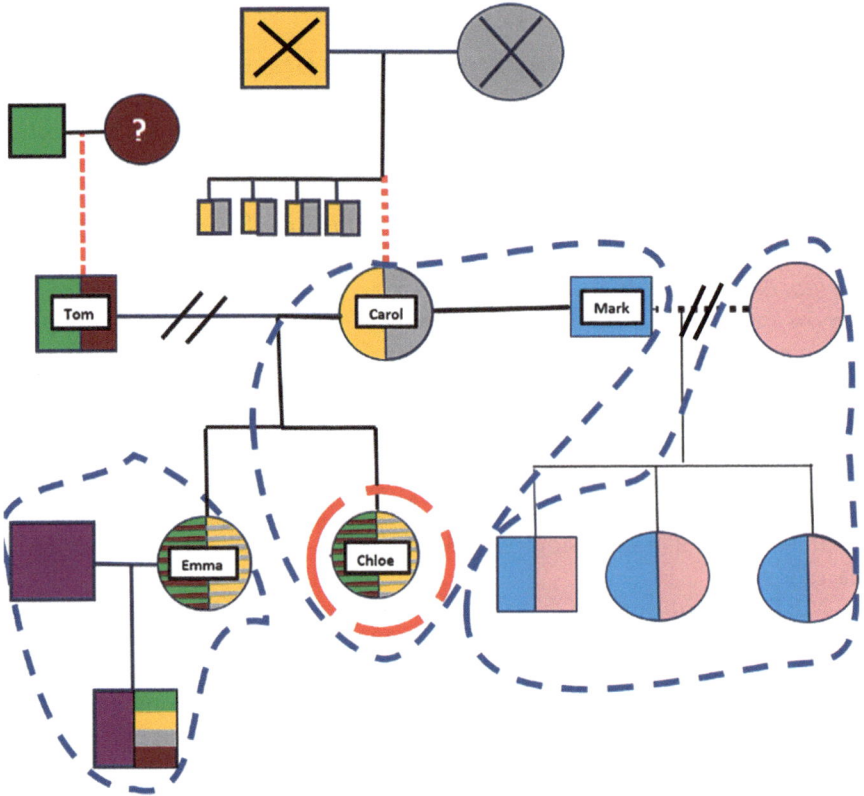

Lives together:	● ● ● ● ● ● ● ● ● ● ● ●	Parent Unkown:	?
Broken relationship:	● ● ● ● ● ● ● ● ● ● ● ●	Male:	▭
Divorced:	—//—	Female:	◯
Deceased	X	Maternal Grandmother and Grandfather	

Fig. 3.3   Family genogram, making sense of Chloe's story

suicidal thoughts or self-harming behaviours have "a good psychosocial assessment and a structured dynamic clinical formulation with a co-produced safety plan".

Herman's 3 stage model of trauma and recovery informs us of assessing and managing symptoms of trauma that need to be prioritised:1 'safety and stability', 'fight and flight' poor self-care, high risk behaviours, revictimisation and dissociation; and setting goals connected to 2 'remembering and grieving' loss and separation (influenced by Bowlby's work) and 3 'reconnecting and integration' (Herman, 1992, 2022).

SOCIAL domain: Chole had missed most of the first two years of Secondary school and lost touch with friendship groups at school and in the neighbourhood. This began at a time when she was transitioning from primary and to secondary school. In socio-economic terms, Mark (stepfather) and Carol proudly told us that he was a carpet-fitter and was never short of work as a painter and decorator, they owned their house and Carol didn't have to work.

SOCIAL assessment and intervention: Chloe's permission and that of her family was sought to approach the school to see what kind of reintegration program might be possible. Chloe was keen to return to school, she was not being bullied, had no learning difficulties and had a good academic report from her primary school. She wanted to go back to school but needed support and courage to return. She was still on the school register, but for reasons unknown she had not come to the attention of the School's Welfare Officer. The School could not have been more accommodating and the pastoral head visited Chloe and her parents at home to devise a support plan and stepped timetable for her return.

COGNITIVE BEHAVIOURAL domain: Chole's thoughts, feelings, physical sensations and actions were seen as key contributors to the development of her mental ill health and feeling trapped in her distress. Although there is significant research including NICE Guidelines for Depression and Anxiety (2022, NG222) to recommend the strengths of CBT; it was agreed that the complexity of SAD, the transgenerational ACEs and trauma may not be addressed fully by a solution focused approach for Chole. The evidence suggests that CBT is effective at treating social anxiety disorder when paired with other treatments (Spence et al., 2000).

COGNITIVE BEHAVIOUR assessment and interventions: Parents were offered CBT informed 'progress meetings' (without Chloe, but with her knowledge) to help them parent and problem solve ways to help Chloe cope at home and encourage her return to school. They included principles of graded exposure to social fears, address negative patterns of thinking, enhancing communication and assertiveness to support lasting improvement (Spence et al., 2000). CBT was an extremely effective intervention to use with the parents. Chloe's metal health improved, she returned to school, and started to make friends and catch up with her missed education. At this point it was important to review the formulation process and think about the overall picture of the other family members. From my clinical experience it was crucial to engage the parents in the solution. They (mother, father and stepfather) had become unsure what to do, preferring to avoid any conversations that might cause stress for Chloe. The progress then enabled us to take a psychoanalytic, trauma informed approach that enables us to question our observations about the unconscious explanations for Chloe's distress. At the start of treatment Chole, her father and stepfather were not aware of her mother Carol's childhood sexual abuse. These were stories that were 'unknown, unheard and untold' until they were 'outed' by Chloe finding and reading her mother's old diaries. The formulation discussion changed course at the point of this new knowledge.

PSYCHOANALYTICAL AND SYSTEMIC DOMAIN

In terms of Psychoanalytic theory we considered Erikson who viewed personality across the lifespan, comprising of eight stages where 'basic conflicts' need to be negotiated by the individual in order to make a healthy emotional transition to the next stage. Progression in terms of chronological age is not a given (Table 3.1, is a summary chart of Erikson's Psychosocial Stages of Development). We can speculate about which were the most polarising basic conflicts for Chole but also what are her strengths and protective factors. For example, Chole met all expected milestones as a toddler, she enjoyed primary school, made friendships and was educationally successful. Staff at the Secondary School were very supportive, helping to devise a plan that gradually invited her participation and socialising back into her peer group in breaktime and educational activity, although for reasons of confidentiality they were not fully conversant with the family history; they appreciated that adolescents need to develop a sense of self and personal identity, the basic emotional conflict being 'identity verses role confusion'; peer relationships being essential to this crucial stage of development.

Erikson's ideas about the first stage of development concern a basic assumption of 'trust versus mistrust' can be thought about in the way that many people struggling with mental health problems, across the lifespan, may experience the world as a dangerous place and it may be that they have had stressful or traumatic experiences that support this fear and affect relationships in later life. This aligns with Bowlby's ideas of building 'a secure base' (Bowlby, 1988, 1993) and should inform our therapeutic stance.

Erikson talks about 'ego diffusion' in adolescents where the individual is struggling to integrate different roles and aspects of the self. When Chole spoke about her feelings of depression and anxiety she could not pinpoint occasions when she was more or less distressed but described being emotionally labile, feeling lost and uncertain. Erikson asserts that adolescence is a second

Table 3.1 Erikson's psychosocial stages: A summary chart

Age	Conflict	Important events	Outcome
Infancy (birth to 18 months)	Trust vs. Mistrust	Feeding	Hope
Early Childhood (2 to 3 years)	Autonomy vs. Shame and Doubt	Toilet Training	Will
Preschool (3 to 5 years)	Initiative vs. Guilt	Exploration	Purpose
School Age (6 to 11 years)	Industry vs. Inferiority	School	Confidence
Adolescence (12 to 18 years)	Identity vs. Role Confusion	Social Relationships	Fidelity
Young Adulthood (19 to 40 years)	Intimacy vs. Isolation	Relationships	Love
Middle Adulthood (40 to 65 years)	Generativity vs. Stagnation	Work and Parenthood	Care
Maturity (65 to death)	Ego Integrity vs. Despair	Reflection on Life	Wisdom

opportunity to negotiate toddlerhood as the basic task is repeated, i.e. exploring the world and our role within it through social relationships.

Listening to the story in relation to risk assessment of suicidality and self-harm Systemic, narrative influences upon formulation when listening to stories of self-harm are articulated in Brown & Kimball's (2012) phenomenological research "Cutting to Live". The authors found three significant categories reported by people who self-harm: self-harm is misunderstood, self-harm has a role, and advice to professionals is *"we're not suicidal, don't judge us and get educated"* (p. 12) clearly the statement 'we are not suicidal' may not be the case for all; however, these strong words implore us to not jump to conclusions and continued professional development. McCabe et al.'s (2023) paper "Asking about self-harm during risk assessments in psychosocial assessment in emergency department: questions that facilitate and deter disclosure of self-harm" highlights the subtle difference between phrasing questions that close down possibilities for disclosure, i.e. assume the person is not planning on further harming behaviours instead we should be styling open questions that invite disclosure mindful that many people who hold ambivalent feelings towards both self-harm and suicidality are at significant risk. The two intentions should therefore not be seen as separate entities but are often enmeshed; open questions therefore significantly influence disclosure and our appreciation of the 'type and strength of someone's thoughts' (2023).

Communication patterns that we observe within families and within the process of formulation, team case discussion can be informative but may need to be challenged. Discursive language and labelling, ways of describing things *as if* it is a truth need to be *held lightly*. The power relationship within formulation should be structured in order of safe practice and the person's need, not which professional voices, family member voices or theories are privileged and held aloft. In this respect it may be necessary to consider 'ontological' (our assumptions about what there is to know) and 'epistemological' reflexivity (how we come to know something), i.e. our knowledge of both are culturally constructed (Finlay & Gough, 2003).

Systemic/Family Therapy informed thinking in formulation: The Social GGRRAAACCEEESSS (Burnham, 2012) and **LUUUTT model** (Pearce & Pearce, 1990) both acronyms that invite us to consider possible aspects of personal and social identity (GENDER; GEOGRAPHY; RACE; RELIGION; AGE; ABILITY; APPEARANCE; CULTURE; CLASS / CASTE; EDUCATION; EMPLOYMENT; ETHNICITY; SPIRITUALITY; SEXUALITY and SEXUAL ORIENTATION).

Social GGRRAAACCEEESSS for Chloe was considered within the context of her mother's ACEs and childhood sexual abuse. Notions of gender, age, attractiveness and education continued to be the dominant narratives and at the forefront of my thinking, questions like what does it mean to be female and becoming a teenager and young woman, and the implications of these changes for and from the perspective of different family members.

The LUUUTT model helps us deconstruct narratives; the stories that we tell, stories that might be told about us and stories that are not known (stories LIVED; UNTOLD; UNKNOWN & UNHEARD subjective stories that may not be conscious; TOLD meaning we make about these stories which may inform aid or inhibit our actions; and in the TELLING the way we tell our stories which can change in the moment and across the life course). We had been working with parental 'story told' (LUUUTT). However, the 'story lived' for Chloe about not going to school was causing her to feel anxious. Chloe also told us that she sometimes worried about her mum and what she would do without her mother if something should happen; separation from her mother was also anxiety provoking. The parents valued education for their daughter, and understood their legal responsibility as parents, but also had their own narratives about school having not been particularly engaged or interested in education when they were of a similar age, and were ambivalent about the benefits. Education had been something to endure and their financial and life successes in adulthood were seen as unrelated.

When working with the family, specifically the parents as a couple, explanation of this model helped frame their understanding and attachment bonds as so eloquently advocated by Johnson's (2002) "Emotionally Focused Couple Therapy with Trauma Survivors" a book that has been so influential in my work as a family therapist. Johnson explains the '*trauma trap*' that "when our bodies and feelings are experienced as being out of control, just being in touch with them seems dangerous" (p. 21). This account is relatable to Chloe's mother having kept secret her abuse, choosing to move away from home, never to return and not being able to speak of trauma until she sought help for herself having seen Chloe's mental health improve. Carol said she was then able to see Chloe 'developing into a young woman'.

The individual work with Chloe became less frequent as she regained her confidence and enjoyment in life. Although there were progress meetings the necessary attachment work was focused with mother and step-father who were courageous in their thinking and engaged in building their relationship.

Formulation discussions returned to thinking about Carol's early years and how profoundly this might have ruptured emotional bonds as a mother and in her adult relationships. Theories of attachment, separation and loss tell us that a primary caregiver's intimate care and touch provides vital physical, emotional and neurobiological regulation in the infant. The reflexive responsibility of the caregiver to provide verbal and non-verbal communications to both sooth (nurture safety and calm distress) and stimulate (social play) cements the infants' capacity to innately turn towards the caregiver. The reciprocity of a healthy relationship helps us to manage risk and unpredictably throughout our lives.

Contemporary practice considers the idea of multiple attachment figures across the lifespan—restorative relationships where we can grow, develop and entrust in the relationship. The capacity to negotiate the good and the bad about oneself is learnt in these early years and reexperienced in friendships for

Chole and in the adult intimate relationship between Carol and Mark. These connections can be underdeveloped or absent when a person experiences abuse or severe trauma, and the psychological development of their identity / personality can become fragmented. Although Carol appeared to be functioning she had disassociated painful memories and found it difficult to have emotional and social relationships. Bradley (2018) explains that fragmentation instinctively causes us to keep some of these pieces hidden but also of the possibility that 'in a safe space or a safe way' we can start to express them. Carol told us in one of the later couples' sessions that "It is not about someone telling you they love you but starting to feeling worthy of being loved".

The role of the clinician is more than attending to physical health care needs. It is the relational involvement with the person's distress by possessing the capacity to contain the suffering by responding appropriately. This is communicated in the compassionate way, clinical tasks starting with assessment are conducted. The clinician holds the person's emotional state in mind the same way Bowlby (1988) writes about the attachment relationship between mother, or other primary caregiver, and the child. Being attuned to the needs and vulnerabilities of the patient while not becoming overwhelmed by them is the necessary shift from empathy to objective professional caring.

Formulation as a Supervisory Tool

Kadushin (1992) states there are three main functions of supervision: educative, supportive and administrative or management function. Hughes and Pengelly (1997) and subsequent authors argue that focusing upon the emotional impact of the work is more important than simply being supportive. I have noted a concerning trend amongst colleague in practice and training institutions to explain away decades of shortcomings and attribute far too much of their own malaise to the Covid-19 pandemic. In order for clinicians to not become hardened and maintain a balanced approach to the possibilities of the care on offer, support needs to be provided and sought through clinical discussion; reflective and reflexive practice; and good management of staff and the care they provide. The process of formulation can garner multidisciplinary critical thinking and feedback to advance a team approach by separating the emotional impact of clinical contact and restore clarity and clinical theory and research informed direction. The 'container' of formulation is therefore as relevant to the efficacy and problem solving capabilities of the clinician and organisation as it is to those we serve and care for. Sharing the burden of decision making, inviting and valuing the contribution of all, and co-creating through consultation with people and carers with lived experience is a fundamental to systemic formulation.

In support of **formulation as a mitigating process for burnout and directionless practice** and a way to rekindle hope, Evans (2014) explains that the compelling lesson learnt from the Francis Report (2013) into serious failings at Mid Staffs Foundation Trust was that the NHS needs to "put the patient first and everything else should flow from there". The Francis report highlighted 290 recommendations in total, many of which are heartbreakingly echoed as failing in subsequent inquiries in other NHS and Private care providers. The intrinsic lack of attention and investment in resources and infostructure continues to be impactful upon staff morale, staff retention, and team working which ultimately compromises quality of care.

Gerada (2022) expressed feelings of 'moral injury' about not being able to do the job / profession that you were training to do and 'betrayal' by the lack of investment in the NHS and Social Care. Although Gerada (General Practitioner) concludes her article with the statement that she would not have chosen any other profession—the call to care, support and safeguard the workforce is clear.

Menzies-Lyth's (1959) observational research, "Social systems as a defence against anxiety" outlines a nursing culture of distancing the nurse from the anxiety provoked by the horrors of the job, fears about managing illness, distress and dying and survival. While Menzies-Lyth understood these to be unhelpful reductive defensive practices that talked about "the hernia in bed 9" rather than an appreciation of the person in physical and psychological distress who may also be a parent, a son or daughter and all aspects of personhood, situations and community. She understood the hierarchy and irreconcilable double-bind position of the profession rather than seeing this as a lack of morality which was articulated in a later paper "Facing the Crisis" (Menzies-Lyth, 1999). She explained that she had originally presented her research saying "today I am going to address you as managers" which triggered outrage as the nurses saw themselves as 'caring professionals' not authoritarian rule drivers. In contemporary practice it is essential to acknowledge that all staff need to be engaged in caring management of their work. The division between executive responsibility and management of the care delivered is everyone's responsibility. It is professionally healthy to acknowledge the inherent anxiety that the work provokes in us and to be reflectively responsive. This aspect of formulation is achieved by consciously drawing upon psychoanalytical and systemic principles.

Formulation can aid the clinician and the service user to shift from hopelessness and procrastination to thinking towards a positive view of their future self. It is crucial in order to maintain the momentum that there isn't a full stop after the activity of formulation but an ongoing process of appreciative inquiry about what is *known* in the present, not a de facto truth of a person's past and present but a reasonable way forward that will need review and evaluation as the picture changes.

This chapter has considered just a few of the different themes that were afforded by the use and revisiting of theories in the process of formulation. It is hoped that themes explored might be helpful in your own formulations. However *hold your hypothesis lightly* and use them to inform your assessment not your truth. Ideas of power and powerlessness need to be contextual in all your thinking as they position the service user and the power differentials between us. Ideas of power can also help us to consider its effects on social opportunity and life choices. Think critically about the sometimes paralysing polarities of 'visible and invisible; voiced and unvoiced' (Burnham, 2012) and what affordances, resources and resilience might the person have. Be systemically relational and culturally connected to what is helpful to think about in relation to your work, and question with openness and sensitivity.

> *A well thought-through plan presented to children with meaning can help them to believe that good experiences can happen in the world and they can be real. If they can arrive at this stage of emotional interpretation with a stronger sense of self, they will be able to make sense of the outside world and, with support, use what is being presented to them positively as they begin to feel more real as a person.* (Bradley, 2018, p. 119)

REFERENCES

American Psychiatric Association. (2013). *Diagnostic and statistical manual of mental disorders* (5th ed.). American Psychiatric Association.

American Psychiatric Association, DSM-5 Task Force. (2013). *Diagnostic and statistical manual of mental disorders: DSM-5™* (5th ed.). American Psychiatric Publishing, Inc. https://doi.org/10.1176/appi.books.9780890425596

Bowlby, J. (1969). *Attachment separation, loss.* Hogarth.

Bowlby, J. (1988). *A secure base—Parent-child attachment and healthy human development.* Routledge.

Bowlby, J. (1993). *A secure base.* Routledge.

Bradley, C. (2018). *Revealing the inner world of traumatised children and young people—An attachment-informed model for assessing emotional needs and treatment.* Jessica Kingsley Publishers.

Brown, T. B., & Kimball, T. (2012). Cutting to live: A phenomenology of self-harm. *Journal of Marital and Family Therapy, 39*(2), 195–208.

Burnham, J. (2012). Developments in the social GGRRAAACCEEESSS: Visible-invisible and voiced-unvoiced. In I.-B. Krause (Ed.), *Culture and reflexivity in systemic psychotherapy: Mutual perspectives.* Karnac.

Clark, C., Classen, C. C., Fourt, A., & Shetty, M. (2015). *Treating the trauma survivor: An essential guide to trauma-informed care.* Routledge.

Dube, S. R., Anda, R. F., Felitti, V. J., Chapman, D. P., Williamson, D. F., & Giles, W. H. (2001). Childhood abuse, household dysfunction, and the risk of attempted suicide throughout the life span: Findings from the adverse childhood experiences study. *JAMA, 286,* 3089–3096.

Erikson, E. H. (1964). *Childhood and society* (2nd ed.). W.W. Norton.

Evans, M. (2014). I'm beyond caring, a response to the Francis Report: The failure of social systems in health care to adequately support nurses and nursing in clinical care of patients. *Psychoanalytical Psychotherapy, 28*(2), 193–210.

Finlay, L., & Gough, B. (2003). *Reflexivity—A practical guide for researchers in health and social sciences.* Blackwell Science Ltd.

Forestier, S., Hazen-Brunet, N., Jarrasse, D., Marq, B., & Meyer, M. (Eds.). (2016). *Chagall—The stained glass windows*. Paulist Press.

Gerada, C. (2022). In my 30 years as a GP, the profession has been horribly eroded. *The Guardian*, February 22.

Herman, J. L. (1992). Complex PTSD: A syndrome in survivors of prolonged and repeated trauma. *Journal of Traumatic Stress, 5*(3), 377–391.

Herman, J. L. (2022). *Trauma and recovery—The aftermath of violence—From domestic abuse to political terror* (4th ed.). Basic Books.

Hughes, L., & Pengelly, P. (1997). *Staff supervision in a turbulent environment: Managing process and task in front-line services*. Jessica Kingsley.

International Classification of Diseases (2019/2021) International Classification of Diseases, Eleventh Revision (ICD-11), World Health Organization https://icd. who.int/browse11

Jawaid, A., Roszkowski, M., & Mansuy, I. M. (2018). Transgenerational epigenetics of traumatic stress. In *Progress in molecular biology and translational science—Neuroepigenetics and mental illness, Volume 158*. Academic Press. www.sciencedirect. com/science/article

Johnson, S. M. (2002). *Emotionally focused couples therapy with trauma survivors: Strengthening attachment bonds*. Guilford Press.

Johnson, L., & Dallos, R. (2014). *Formulation in psychology and psychotherapy: Making sense of people's problems* (2nd ed.). Routledge.

Kadushin, A. (1992). *Supervision in social work* (3rd ed.). Columbia University Press.

Kadushin, A. (2002). *Supervision in social work*. Columbia University Press.

Kessler, R. C., McLaughlin, K. A., Green, J. G., et al. (2010). Childhood adversities and adult psychopathology in the WHO World Mental Health Surveys. *British Journal of Psychiatry, 197*, 378–385.

McCabe, R., Bergen, C., Lomas, M., Ryan, M., & Albert, R. (2023). Asking about self-harm during risk assessment in psychosocial assessments in the emergency department: Questions that facilitate and deter disclosure of self-harm. *British Journal of Psychiatry*. https://doi.org/10.1192/bjo.2023.32. Published online by Cambridge University Press.

Menzies-Lyth, I. (1959). Social systems as a defence against anxiety. Reprinted (1998) in *Containing anxiety in institutions* (Vols. 1 and 2, pp. 43–85). Free Association Books.

Menzies-Lyth, I. (1999). Facing the crisis. *Psychoanalytical Psychotherapy, 13*(3), 207–212.

National Confidential Enquiry into Patient Outcome and Death. (2017). *Treat as One*. London. In RCP (2020). *Side by side: A UK-wide consensus statement on working together to help patients with mental health needs in acute hospitals*.

National Institute of Health and Care Excellence. (2022). *Self-harm: Assessment, management and preventing recurrence* (NICE, NG225). www.nice.org.uk/guidance/ng225

National Scientific Council on the Developing Child. (2010). *Early experiences can alter gene expression and affect long-term development*. Working Paper No. 10. www.developingchild.harvard.edu

Oral, R., Ramirez, M., Coohey, C., Nakada, S., Walz, A., Benoit, J., & Peek-Asa, C. (2010). Adverse childhood experiences and trauma informed care: The future of health care. *Pediatric Research, 79*(1), 227–233.

Oxford English Dictionary. (2023). www.oed.com

Pearce, W. B., & Pearce, K. A. (1990). Transcendent storytelling: Abilities for systemic practitioners and their clients. *Human Systems, 9*(3–4), 167–185.

Peters, S. W. (2020). Case formulation and intervention: Application of the five P's framework in substance use counselling. *The Professional Counselor, 10*(3), 327–336.

Royal College of Psychiatry. (2020). Side by side: A UK-wide consensus statement on working together to help patients with mental health needs in acute hospitals. www.rcpsych.ac.uk/docs/default-source/members/faculties/liaison-psychiatry/liaison-sidebyside.pdf

Royal College of Psychiatry. (2023). *Inaccurate suicide risk assessments could be putting lives at risk*. RCP Press Release.

Siegel, D. J. (2020). *The developing mind—How relationships and the brain interact to shape who we are* (3rd ed.). Guilford Press.

Sisk, C. L., & Romeo, R. D. (2019). *Coming of age: The neurobiology and psychobiology of puberty and adolescence*. Oxford University Press.

Spence, S. H., Donovan, C., & Brechman-Toussaint, M. (2000). The treatment of childhood social phobia: The effectiveness of a social skills training-based, cognitive-behavioural intervention, with and without parental involvement. *Journal of Child Psychology and Psychiatry, 41*(6), 713–726. https://doi.org/10.1111/1469-7610.00659

The Lancet Psychiatry. (2022). *Editorial, Vol. 9*. p. 759.

Tully, J., Bhugra, D., Lewis, S. J., Drennan, G., & Markham, S. (2021). Is PTSD over-diagnoses? *The British Medical Journal, 373*(787). https://doi.org/10.1136/bmj.n787

Sources of Help

https://www.gov.scot/publications/trauma-informed-practice-toolkit-scotland/
www.harmless.org.uk
www.mind.org (for over 18s only)
www.rcpsych.ac.uk/helathadvice/parentsandyouthinfor/parentscarers/self-harm.aspx
www.rethink.org
www.samaritans.org
www.youngminds.org.uk

Formulating Distress in Adults and Children Experiencing Physical and Mental Health Problems

Jane Peirson, Claire Grainger, and Georgia Grainger

> **Key Learning Points**
> - Exploring childhood and adulthood experiences of physical health conditions and impacts on mental health
> - The importance of listening and trying to understand how complex physical health challenges impact on the individual, family, friends and social situations
> - Receiving empathy and compassion from professionals is instrumental for hope and feeling valued and understood
> - The co-ordination of care is key

INTRODUCTION

What are the impacts of physical health problems upon the person's mental health? There is no easy answer to this as there are lots of things that can impact. These vary from person to person and every person's experience will be

J. Peirson (✉)
York St John University, York, UK
e-mail: j.peirson@yorksj.ac.uk

C. Grainger
Rotherham, Doncaster and South Humber NHS Trust, Doncaster, UK

G. Grainger
Doncaster, UK

unique to them. This chapter will look at the impacts of some of these factors on the child and adult using the experiences of a person who has grown up with physical and mental health problems throughout childhood and into adulthood. Using the person's case study, the main times of distress will be formulated to understand the impact that situations have had on the person's mental health and physical health, alongside biopsychosocial concepts.

BACKGROUND AND CURRENT THINKING

People with a combination of a serious mental illness and physical health problems have an increased rate of mortality (NHS England, 2023), dying on average 15 to 20 years earlier than the general population. The extent of these issues has been recognised for over a decade, for example in 2012 within an estimated 30 million people with a physical health problem in the UK, 4 million of these people also had mental health problems (Naylor et al., 2012). This can be a cyclical process that is self-fulfilling and it can be hard to determine which has the greater impact upon the person's health and wellbeing outcomes. So, for example it may be that someone has a diagnosis of diabetes; the person feels singled out because they need to be regularly monitoring their blood glucose levels and they need to eat at regular intervals. The fluctuation in their glucose levels also affects their mood and energy levels. The diabetes might have an impact upon other health conditions also, making them more at risk of vision problems, thyroid problems and developing celiac disease. In a child this makes them different to other children. They might miss school for monitoring appointments, miss out on certain activities or need them to be altered to be able to participate which again singles them out as different. These effects of diabetes may have an impact upon the person's mental health as they may be feeling isolated and low in mood. This might mean that they have a loss of appetite, have sleep problems which then have a big impact upon the stability of the person's diabetes. This may then make them feel lethargic, less willing to engage and therefore increase their isolation, which in turn increases their depression, and so the cycle continues. Using formulation can help the person with an understanding of their situation and signs/symptoms, identifying the skills, resources and pathway for prevention/recovery that can help.

The cost to the NHS for people with complex health needs (multiple health needs) is significant (increased costs of 45% for each individual) (Naylor et al., 2012) as is the wider costs to society (such as, higher rates of sick days, lower rates of employment, family members being "informal" carer(s) meaning less contribution to the economy in terms of taxation but higher health needs of their own due to stress factors, etc.). Research by the Kings Fund (Naylor et al., 2012) looking at the co-morbidity of physical health and mental health showed that people with a mental health disorder increased with the number of physical health conditions they had. This is something that within all services in everyday practice is identified as paramount. All services need to have knowledge of the impact of physical health needs upon the person's mental health and vice versa. This has been reflected within nurse education with the introduction of the future nurse standards (NMC, 2018), ensuring that all nurses have a shared awareness of both physical health and mental health.

CURRENT RECOMMENDATIONS FOR TREATMENT OF PEOPLE WITH MENTAL HEALTH AND PHYSICAL HEALTH PROBLEMS

NICE (2009, 2011) advocate for "active case finding" among people with long-term physical health conditions in order to detect mental health problems. This is part of the prevention and early intervention in mental health strategy. By seeking out any early warning signs, interventions can be put in place to prevent these becoming a problem for the person. They recommend services such as Cognitive or Dialectical Behavioural Therapy (CBT/DBT) to help people to understand their problems and deal with them using "talking and behavioural therapies" rather than the complexities of poly-pharmacological interventions. There are also many self-help approaches which can be used to normalise the discussion of mental and emotional aspects of physical illness, and help to target and change unhelpful behaviour patterns. Peer support and self-management programmes are also helpful to increase motivation and inclusivity to reduce isolation, with a need for more social prescribing (look at social work policy and framework).

There is a need to integrate treatment of both mental health and physical health, rather than layering treatment for mild to moderate illnesses and referral to specialist services for complex treatment, to prevent missing the "whole person care" that is required. There are some difficulties in the implementation of this such as considerations over payment, for example it is different funding for mental health and physical health as they are commissioned separately leading to confusion over who would pay for these services. Mental health liaison services in physical health acute settings provide some bridging of the gap in the needs of integrative services. However, they still face difficulties such as different trusts having different commissioning and services and the complications of differing electronic records systems between mental health teams and physical health teams in both primary and secondary care.

Public Health England (2018) describe health inequalities as "avoidable and unfair differences in health status between groups of people or communities". The issue of inequalities is very heavily debated within global politics. UK Parliament (Bunn, 2021) explained that "Mental health inequalities are closely linked to increased risk of having a preventable physical health condition or are themselves caused by other physical conditions. Rising prevalence of non-communicable diseases and conditions (such as type 2 diabetes, cardiovascular disease, some cancers, and neurodegenerative conditions) are a particular concern, as is the increasing prevalence of people developing multiple long-term conditions, across both physical and mental health".

Measuring of heath inequalities in society is a widely contested area. This is due to the many impacting factors that contribute to a person's health, these could include for example:—financial implications, living in deprivation, coping strategies, emotional resilience, access to services, education, employment, etc. The impacting factors are so variable from person to person that using a model to support assessment of these can be useful. A widely used model is Dahlgren and Whitehead (1991) Social Determinants of Health (Fig. 4.1). This model keeps the person at the centre and the impacting factors in an ascending rainbow. It identifies different influences upon the person that might impact upon the person's health needs. Utilising a model such as this can help to focus the assessment of these areas for the person, helping to identify any needs/impacts within these areas—thus, facilitating the opportunity to work with the individual to then formulate what these impacts mean to them. A criticism of using a model for assessment is the rigidity of them, therefore it is worth remembering as in any assessment, that there is a need to remain fluid in the assessment as the needs identified can fluctuate depending on the person's circumstances at the time.

To capture and further expand upon some of the issues identified, a case study will be used. The case study is Georgia's story. Georgia is now an adult and has used her words to tell her story. This is important when working towards a formulation with someone as it keeps it meaningful to the person. It is the role of the practitioner to make steps to understand the person's journey, it is not for the person to try and fit into the agenda of the practitioner. This is then put together to formulate what the impacts of different parts of her life have meant on her psychological wellbeing and physical health. As the formulation is Georgia's own words and it is her formulation, Georgia has been

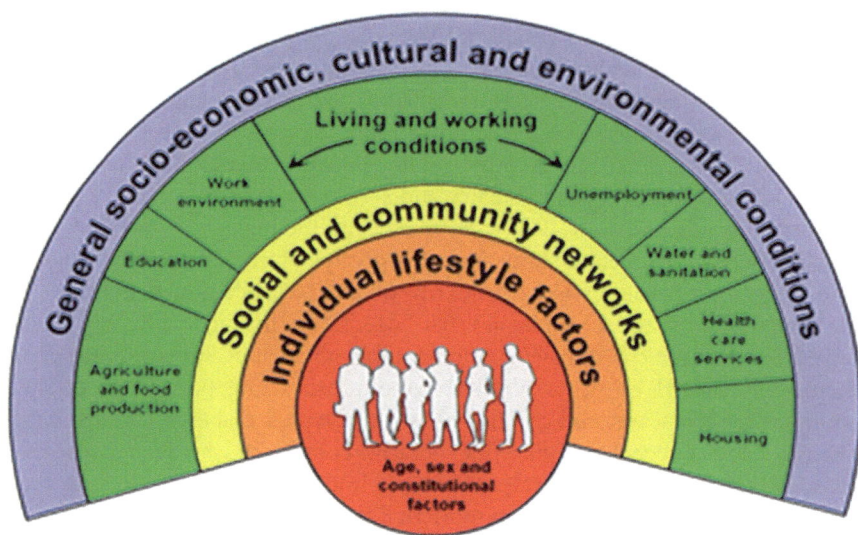

Fig. 4.1 Dahlgren and Whitehead Model (1991) (Replicated with permission from the Institute for Futures Studies)

named as an author on this chapter. Georgia's parents have also contributed to the chapter from their experiences as they are significant in supporting Georgia and advocating for her care. Georgia and her family have all consented to their information being shared within this chapter and to be within the public arena. Georgia has provided a summary of the importance of this to her at the end of the formulation.

GEORGIA'S STORY

Georgia is the first child, her parents underwent fertility treatment to be able to conceive, so she was very much wanted and planned.

When Georgia was born, she arrived 2 weeks early, she was initially healthy, and was discharged home within 2 days.

Georgia was around 6 weeks old when her parents first realised something wasn't right. She had already contracted an infection/pneumonia at age 4 weeks and was still struggling with feeding and swallowing. At 6 weeks she stopped breathing and an ambulance was called. She was taken to resus and admitted. Initially they said it was an ongoing chest infection and she was put on IV antibiotics. She improved and was discharged home.

Georgia's mother states: *"As you can imagine, being first time parents, this was very scary to us. At the first admission staff made us feel very safe and reassured, but did imply we were anxious as we were new to parenting."*

Following this first episode, Georgia continued to struggle with her breathing, and was admitted over 4 times before she was 10 weeks old. Each admission was due to breathing difficulties and infections.

This continued until she was around 4 months old, when she stopped breathing again. This time she was blue-lighted back into hospital, and Georgia's mother states as parents they felt useless. They were scared and worried that they may lose their baby girl. Each admission, Georgia was managed symptomatically, but no further investigations were made and this was very frustrating to the parents.

Georgia's mother says: *"However, it was at this point (4 months of age) we met Dr K (paediatric consultant). He asked us to allow him to investigate Georgia's health and investigate why this kept happening."*

This is when the investigations started, genetic tests were undertaken which showed Georgia had very poor head control and was described as a floppy baby. This had never been picked up on previous admissions or by the midwives/health visitors.

It was around 6 months of age that it was found Georgia had a chromosomal disorder and additional tests were instigated to look at muscle weakness. She also had hydrocephaly, sleep apnea and very little immune system at this time, and this required close monitoring.

It was around 9 months of age that Georgia was sent to neurology for further investigations for myopathy, as she remained very floppy, unable to crawl and still struggled to hold her head.

An autism diagnosis came at age 3 years.

Tonsils and adenoids were removed at age 3.5 years, to help with the management of sleep apnea. Georgia was prescribed prophylaxis antibiotics from the age of 1 year until around age 9, to help minimise this risk of infection. A scoliosis diagnosis came later, at around age 13. This had been missed due to her myopathy masking the presentation.

Georgia has always struggled with her hearing which has required multiple surgeries.

The family were initially prepared for the worst with Georgia. The specialist said that the likely outcome for Georgia would be that she would have moderate learning needs, would never walk, and may struggle to communicate—when in fact this is not the case.

Georgia now has multiple diagnoses of Duplication Chromosomal Translocation 7q 11.13 associated with hypotonia and Asperger's Syndrome, Myopathy, Chromosome Translocation 22q 11T, Ehlers Danlos (Vascular), Connective Tissue Disorder, Scoliosis (moderate), Bilateral Hearing Loss, Immuno-suppression, Hypogammaglobulinemia with recurrent pulmonary infections. This means that she endures a lot of pain and discomfort in her everyday life which also affects her mental health and wellbeing.

Using Georgia's own words and input from her mother (family perspective), the following section will look at formulating Georgia's physical health impacts upon her mental health through different experiences in her lifespan.

Describe a time when you (Georgia) feel your physical health has impacted on your lifestyle…

"When I have to cancel/adapt plans because I am in significant pain—this prevents me from going out with friends. I have never been able to go and do what others take for granted, such as bike riding, ice skating or just something simple like playing on the park as I haven't got the strength or balance to allow me to do this.

Having to stay home from university/school due to chronic pain and fatigue, missing out on lectures and building friendships, as I am limited in what I can do.

An example when I was in school: I was sat in science when my knee decided to dislocate—the pain was excruciating, and I screamed out loud because of this. The whole class had to be removed, and an ambulance called, which took a while to arrive. During this time other pupils and friends continued to look in to see what was happening. Following this incident other students including friends were very wary, asking me questions and some even called me a freak. Following this dislocation, I was on crutches, and again this prevented me from attending regular classes, as some were upstairs—it stopped me from being with peers and friends during this time. I dislocate easily, due to my condition, which is associated with Ehlers Danlos and Connective Tissue Disorder. I continue to dislocate my shoulder now and again and this leads to chronic pain and at least 6-8 week recovery times."

How did it make you feel?

"Selfish

A burden to others

Embarrassed, ashamed of what people thought

Different to others

Scared, I continually worry about my knees and shoulders dislocating. I experience chronic pain daily and this is something I am trying to manage, but it makes me upset, and angry and frustrated, as I just want it to go away.

I struggle with anxiety and constantly worry about what other people think of me—the hardest part is my disabilities are not always visible, and others often don't understand my illness, which again leads to me feeling alone and isolated at times."

What was happening before the situation occurred? Was there anything in particular that was different about that day or the time that led up to the situation?

"My pain and chronic fatigue is ongoing, it's something I'm having to learn to live with and manage daily. I know that if I walk too much or do too much in one day, the impact on my body the next day is significant—for example, if I go for a short walk, or shopping to my local town, the next day I will be limited in what I can do. It often leaves me lying in bed, taking extra pain meds and recovering—again this leads to many mixed emotions for me, as it makes me feel like I can't do things like others do. I can become very tearful but angry at the same time, but now I am older I am starting to manage this better and I feel I am aware of my limitations.

Thinking around day to day tasks, I have to pre-plan and think about what I am doing, who I'm doing it with and who will be there to support me if needed—and this can be a task in itself."

What happened at the time, what did you do? How did it make you feel?

"When I dislocated my knee, it was very difficult, as all I could do was sit there, as I couldn't move. Teachers didn't know what to do, it took over 2 hours for paramedics to come, but once my mum arrived from work, I felt more reassured, as she knows how to calm me down—my dad also came and this helped. I felt stupid at the time, knowing others/friends had seen what happened. I felt embarrassed and like the teachers didn't believe me at first. They kept telling me to get up and tried to move me. It wasn't until my mum spoke to them over the phone and directed them in what to do that, they left me in the classroom. I was prescribed a medication called Buccal Midazolam, a relaxant that would help my knee slip back into place, and this was a treatment I had used many times and had found useful, but staff in school weren't trained to administer it, as there were no community services that had capacity to train staff at that time."

What did you do after the situation? Was that helpful at the time? What about in the long run?

"After, I had to take time off school, I retuned but was in a wheelchair and had to use crutches for quite some time. This wasn't anything new to me, as I have a wheelchair and crutches that I have to use intermittently due to my ongoing health needs/condition. School were very supportive of me, but again, it made me feel different to others, when staff would fuss around me, and it put friends off wanting to spend time with me."

What is important to you that helps when you feel frustrated?

"Talking with my mum and dad, and one friend in particular that experiences similar issues. Knowing that I have a supportive family around me, and teachers/lecturers that understand me. Having a wheelchair and aids I can use to keep me mobile when needed."

Are there any significant times in your life when you have felt that you are unable to do things that your friends/peers are doing? How does that make you feel?

"I can't ride a bike; I only drive an automatic car and struggle with walking long distances and fall frequently—this is due to my myopathy, pain, Elders Danlos etc. These things make me feel embarrassed and it annoys me when people ask why as they don't understand, nor do I feel comfortable trying to explain it to others. I struggle when communicating with others and this is linked to my autism, so I can find it even harder than others when people don't understand."

We can see from Georgia's interview that there are a lot of factors here that have led to the way in which she is feeling. We can use the principles of the 4Ps (predisposing factors, precipitating factors, perpetuating factors and protective factors (Johnstone & Dallos, 2014) with the biopsychosocial model (Engel, 1977) to help understand this. Table 4.1 presents an example of using the bio-psychosocial 4Ps approach to formulation for Georgia's case study (adapted from Barker (1995) and the Weerasekera (1993), formulation models available online from the PsychDB website (PsychDB 2024). This is a good formulation model for Georgia's case study as the biopsychosocial approach to care recognises the three different domains of health: biological, psychological and sociological; and their relationship to each other whilst being able to capture the person's experience. By breaking the three domains down into the 4Ps approach this enables the person and the practitioner to be able to see the impacting factors of each area and how they relate and feed into the following area. So, for example being able to see that the predisposing factors lead to the precipitating and then the perpetuating factors—this model then suggests that by breaking it down into the biological first, then the sociological it is then possible to see how these elements have impacted the psychological wellbeing of the person. Then by using this understanding and the protective factors there is a starting point for thinking about a strengths-based approach to the person's journey to understanding and managing their psychological wellbeing (such as a wellness recovery action plan (WRAP) (Copeland, 2002).

ANGER AND FRUSTRATION

Georgia describes feelings of anger and frustration about her situation. Communication difficulty is one of the main factors that contribute to frustration which can result in anger and/or aggression. People with physical health problems often report feelings of frustration at not being able to express their health problems and not being understood or heard. This is apparent in Georgia's situation in the way that she had the diagnosis that school were

Table 4.1 Biopsychosocial 4Ps formulation

4Ps of formulation	Biological	Psychological	Sociological
Predisposing	Premature birth Infection/pneumonia at 4 weeks Stopped breathing at 6 weeks (chest infection) Repeated admissions for breathing difficulties and infections, further episode of stopping breathing Poor head control, floppy baby Genetic testing at 4 months 6 months—chromosomal disorder, muscle weakness, hydrocephaly, sleep apnea, poor immunity 9 months—Myopathy 3 years—Autism diagnosis 3.5 years tonsils and adenoids removed to help with sleep apnea 1–9 years prescribed prophylaxis antibiotics due to infection risk 13 years Scoliosis Hearing difficulties and numerous surgeries for this. Multiple diagnoses: Duplicate Chromosomal Translocation 7q 11.13 associated with: hypotonia and Asperger's syndrome, Myopathy, Chromosome translocation 22q 11T, Ehlers Danlos (Vascular), Connective tissue disorder, Scoliosis (moderate), Bilateral hearing loss, Immuno-suppression, Hypogammaglobulinemia with recurrent pulmonary infections.	Being different from the other children Being singled out (example of knee dislocation) Feeling stupid—unable to do anything Good role modelling from parents Secure attachment style with parents but due to Autism traits difficult to understand other people's responses and difficulties with communicating with others, this effects relationships with friends	First child Supportive parents Has one sibling—sister Stable family lifestyle—both parents employed Difficult making friendships in school Missed time in school due to health and appointments

(continued)

Table 4.1 (continued)

4Ps of formulation	Biological	Psychological	Sociological
Precipitating	Unable to do things others do due to poor strength and balance Knee dislocation at school, as an example of a significant traumatic event. (There were many other examples.) Needing to use wheelchair or crutches to aid mobility Poor sleep due to pain and sleep apnea	Repeated experiences resulting in the following psychological feelings and behaviours: Selfish Burden Embarrassed Ashamed Different Scared Angry Upset Frustrated	Cancelling plans Unable to do things that others do—bike riding, ice skating, playing in the park Missing lectures Missing opportunities with friends and struggling to build friendships due to health Teaching staff not trained to use the medication that helped (with dislocations) and no community services that had capacity to train staff Staff fusing around put friends off wanting to spend time with you The repeating of these situations as they are out of your control due to your health
Perpetuating	Chronic PAIN and discomfort Autism affects relationships FATIGUE Dislocation on joints These are chronic issues that do not stop Not offered any psychological support (until adulthood for pain management)	Anxiety and worry of what other people think of you—these have been reinforced over childhood experiences Your disabilities are not always visible—people do not understand Adult health services do not understand you Isolated and alone (at times) You struggle to try and explain to others, and also don't want to explain to others repeatedly Struggle to communicate with others (your needs) linked to your autism Feeling lost and unheard Knocked confidence when not heard Attachment with family remains secure, however still struggles with building relationships with others	Continuing to need time off, missing out on making friends No one in services to co-ordinate care now in adult services • FROM FAMILY PERSPECTIVE: Will Georgia ever experience a different type of love (i.e. with a partner) Will Georgia ever experience a fully independent life—how will that impact on full-time employment, finances, living in her own home, etc.…

Protective	FAMILY—genetic conditions	FAMILY—know how to calm you down	GREAT FAMILY SUPPORT
	More aware of your own limitations	You now plan your day-to-day activities (though this can be exhausting and timely)	Family to continue to be an advocate and fight for the services needed
	More aware of your abilities	You plan now who is around to support if needed	One friend with similar needs that understands
	Having wheelchair and aids that you can use when needed	Staff/work colleagues around that understand your needs	Good GP
	Pain management—Health psychology sessions helpful and independently accessed	• FROM FAMILY PERSPECTIVE:	Despite the missed time in education, you have achieved your degree!!!
		Resilient	
		Determination	
		Amazing personality	
		Strong, independent, proved everyone wrong!	

aware of, but they did not know how to deal with the situation. There was a lack of community services in which to support her in her school environment.

Some people who are in pain can show signs of anger and/or aggression. This can be due to differing factors such as neurological changes, and expressions of feelings that are not being understood or may not be able to be articulated. This can be a problem in children (especially the very young, or people with communication difficulties) when they do not have the vocabulary or cognition to be able to express themselves. A study by Niel et al. (2007) identified that the more pain tolerated by their study participants, the sooner they tended to initiate aggression. These are similar findings to research looking into the association of pain and aggression in patients that have dementia, especially when they are unable to communicate their pain (Sampson et al., 2015). These findings can be transferred to people that experience ongoing (or chronic) pain due to their physical health problems, especially if they are feeling that they are unheard with regard to their pain, helping us to understand why the pain response can show anger and/or aggression and/or frustration as in Georgia's case.

Depending on the person's developed coping mechanisms these can play a contributing part in the display of anger and aggression. People that have not developed differing ways of coping with their health issues/needs may use anger or aggression as a way of coping with these issues/needs this is sometimes seen in children that have experienced trauma (McCrory et al., 2024). Though these are often seen as "negative" coping mechanisms, for some people these are the only ways that they have in managing; for example, the bodily responses to aggression (hyper arousal from chemical changes in the brain creating the fight or flight response). These might be sufficient to help alleviate the situation that the person finds themselves in at that time, even though this may be through demonstrating anger or aggression.

By helping someone to identify why they are feeling frustrated and angry is the first step in helping them to develop strategies to manage this.

LONELINESS AND ISOLATION

We can clearly see from Georgia's experience here that having to be removed from the environment with her experience at school had led to further feelings of "selfishness" and being different to her peers. These kinds of examples lead to feelings of guilt and shame, and due to not wanting to be seen like this can lead to someone wanting to self-isolate and therefore experience feelings of loneliness.

Loneliness and isolation have a negative effect on mental health, increasing symptoms of low mood and anxiety. These might include physical responses like poor diet, increased feelings of panic and sleep disturbance which can then impact upon physical health again enabling the cyclical nature of these difficulties.

The Campaign to End Loneliness (2022) suggests that there were approximately 49.63% of adults (25.99 million people) in the UK living with loneliness or isolation. The Office for National Statistics (2018) suggests that there are 11.3% of children aged 10 to 15 years, and 9.8% of young adults aged 16 to 24 years that are living with loneliness and isolation. The data during the Covid pandemic has not yet been collated but this is expected to have increased in children and young adults due to Covid restrictions particularly for people that are clinically vulnerable due to physical health problems. Isolation and loneliness can be a significant problem for people with mental health and physical health problems. This may be due to the individual's actual abilities to be involved in certain activities due to health restrictions or from other reasons such as a lack of understanding or stigma from others.

People that experience hostility due to prejudice or bullying may feel isolation and loneliness. People with special education needs or a disability are twice as likely to experience prejudice or bullying (Anti-Bullying Alliance, 2016). The causes for this are often varied, however one school of thought is due to the lack of understanding and fear of what the person does not understand. People often avoid talking to the person about health conditions that they do not understand which can lead to further feelings of isolation for that person. Friendship groups are established by finding people that have common features or characteristics. This is often difficult for people experiencing isolation due to their health needs.

SPIRITUALITY

Spirituality is important for everyone and in times of distress is significant, yet it is something that is often forgotten about or lacking in understanding. Spirituality is often confused with religion, and though it can sometimes include religious beliefs this is not always the case. Spirituality is about the person's values, what is important to them and why. The importance of recognising someone's spiritual needs can be traced back to Florence Nightingale, when she recognised that attending to someone's physical health needs alone was not enough to aid their recovery, and that the holistic approach to care was required including their spirituality (Macrae, 1995). Spirituality is about recognising the hope, meaning and purpose of the person's life and without these the person can lose their sense of worth and self-aspirations. Spirituality is very personal and sensitive to a person and they may be very reluctant to share this, or sometimes it may be difficult for the person to recognise what this actually is to them. Hence, to discover this with a person, the communication and spending time to build the therapeutic relationship is significantly important here.

Spirituality often underpins the person's views, values and beliefs on some medical conditions and treatment of them, both for their physical health and their mental health. For example, some Nigerian cultures have beliefs about some mental health conditions being caused by supernatural causes, witchcraft or possession of evil spirits (Labinjo et al., 2020). Another example is some religious cultures' views on contraception, abortion and blood transfusions etc. Having an understanding of the person's beliefs and values helps practitioners in understanding the person and how to provide best care in line with the person's spiritual needs. Working with someone's spiritual needs can cause internal conflict for the practitioner especially if they are conflicting with the practitioner's spirituality. This is something the practitioner needs to have self-awareness about and develop support and supervision structures to enable them to work through these to prevent emotional burnout, but also to prevent trying to instil their own spiritual beliefs on the person they are working with. Ruth Stoll's work (Stoll, 1979) was pivotal in providing some guidelines in assessing spirituality, and many have since then attempted to further develop this work. The Office for Health Improvement and Disparities (2021) provides government guidance on working with people's culture, spirituality and religion. However, a universal assessment on how to carry out an assessment of the spirituality of a person is still debated and not clearly defined and it is usually practitioners' skills and experience that determine how the assessment is formulated.

To demonstrate why spirituality is important we can identify from Georgia's case study that the support that is around her is key to her wellbeing. She has explained that what helps her the most when feeling unwell with either her physical or mental health is feeling safe and loved. This is important to be aware of as it helps to plan how to best support Georgia throughout her life. For example, when Georgia needs to go into a new work setting, having someone that understands her needs is going to be significant. Or if she needs to attend hospital, then having her family around is going to significantly decrease her levels of distress. This can also help Georgia to communicate what is going on in her care, with her family member also acting as an advocate for Georgia.

Trauma

Trauma has different definitions for different types of experiences, for example the Oxford Dictionary definition describes trauma as *"caused by severe shock, stress or fear, especially when the harmful effects last for a long time"*. The Cambridge Dictionary describes it as *"severe and lasting emotional shock and pain caused by an extremely upsetting experience, or a case of such shock happening"* or *"physical injury, usually caused by an accident or attack, or a case of such injury happening"*. The message here is that when we are talking about trauma it is something that is unique to the person that has experienced it.

Felitti et al. (1998) conducted the first ground-breaking study for Kaiser Permanente health care organisation which started in 1995, into the impact of Adverse Childhood Experiences (ACEs) on adulthood health, identifying the relationship between childhood events and adulthood poor health outcomes. Since the initial study there has been more research completed and the evidence of poorer outcomes in both mental health and physical health is well evidenced and documented (Asmussen et al., 2020; World Health Organisation, 2021). The terms and understanding of what now contributes to an "ACE" is much more expansive and is generally accepted to be anything that causes the child to experience a "traumatic" response as defined above.

Working with the person in understanding their trauma, the impact that this has had upon them from the individual's perspective, then using this with the identified skills of the person to help formulate understanding and coping skills/strategies, are the basics of recovery and working in a trauma informed way (Harris & Fallot, 2001; Sweeney & Taggart, 2018). Trauma informed care is a key model that is followed in mental health nursing, and an objective of the NHS Long Term Plan (2019). Trauma informed care's key principles are the promotion of safety for the person and putting interventions in place to promote safety. The message is conveyed that staff are trustworthy—they do what they say they will in an open and honest, transparent way. People are given an informed choice in their care and practitioners work in collaboration with the person, empowering them. As previously discussed, people are recognised and treated with respect in line with their cultural considerations. It is an effective way of working with all people, regardless of if they have experienced a traumatic event. Listening to the person's narrative, "what have you been through", "what is your story" rather than asking "what is wrong with you?", which has connotations of blame, or is a narrow focus of looking at one specific area rather than the whole person. It is a timely way of working, one that requires the practitioner to work at building the therapeutic relationship and prioritising listening to the person. With many competing factors on staff time and prioritising therapeutic interventions, it may be helpful for staff to reflect if they are incorporating trauma-informed outlooks. If it is not delivered correctly, it is ineffective and risks alienating people from accessing services (Sweeney & Taggart, 2018). This approach is very effective in supporting people that have endured ACEs, but if staff are not understanding the impact of ACEs upon the child/person (as identified above) it raises the questions of how effective that treatment is in meeting their needs. As we will see from Georgia's case study that at times through her care, particularly since her move into adult services, the focus has often changed from a person-centred trauma informed approach to a more singularly focussed approach, usually on one aspect of her physical health. This has made her feel very frustrated, not listened to and not able to navigate the complexities of adult care services.

How did the support and health services that Georgia received impact upon her mental health and wellbeing?

Formulating care with the distressed person is an excellent method of helping the person to gain an understanding and clarity of a complex situation, but when there are multiple co-morbidities the need for group team formulation may be helpful (Hartley, 2021). When the impacting factors for someone's health needs are complex, an understanding of the different aspects, roles and responsibilities and shared understanding of the person's care is essential. In Georgia's case this is something that happened better in children's services but less so in adult services. There are many impacting factors for this, often due to overstretched services, lack of time and resources to be available for complex meetings, etc. However, this is short-sighted. If better care and intervention is implemented in the short term, then the improvement in people's health is felt long term and therefore reduces the detrimental impact on services long term (both physical and mental health).

How do you feel about the services that you receive?

Georgia: *"I often feel as if some services aren't doing enough to help me—especially now I'm older. Since leaving children's services due to turning 19, no one coordinates my care—I have multiple appointments with different specialists, such as Cardiology, Orthopaedics and Neurology—but they don't speak to each other. They rely solely on me approaching them and without my parents I wouldn't be able to do this due to my anxiety. I feel like it's a constant battle to be heard, and that no one really cares about how I feel, as they don't really understand me and disabilities."*

Do they work together? How do they communicate with each other?

Georgia: *"When I was younger, so from being born, I was under the care of a community paediatrician Dr K who coordinated all of my care as I was under many different specialists. He would hold regular MDT (multidisciplinary team) meetings, to ensure all services were working together and had the same goals and outcomes. I looked forward to seeing him. He stayed with me until handing over my care when I was nearly 20 years old. He is someone I will never forget. But as I said earlier, the moment I transitioned to adult services, I felt lost, unheard and alone. My mum and dad had to fight for services to be involved, but thankfully I have a supportive GP who has also known me since being a very small child. He will often support mum when services are required."*

Do different services understand your health needs well?

"Not now, as I said above—But when I was under children's they most certainly did. I was under different children's hospitals and they would all regularly meet to discuss my case and needs, they also included my mum and dad in this, as they understood my needs and were able to be my voice when needed."

Do they understand who you are as a person? Is that important to you when you are accessing services?

"It is important that they understand who I am as a person, but I don't think they do any more—I still need my mum to come to appointments with me, and they will often speak to her rather than me and this makes me feel as if they think I am unable to understand what they are saying. They will ask what I need, but don't really see me for who I am. They don't understand the impact my health needs and neurodiversity needs have on my daily living skills and emotional health."

Now that you are an adult do the services come through you or does your mum still co-ordinate care? How difficult is that? How do you feel about organising your care (if applicable)?

"As mentioned, I still need my mum to come to appointments with me, and often she also arranges appointments and contacts health services on my behalf. I would like to do this on my own but feel my voice is unheard, and this knocks my confidence massively. I also get anxious when speaking on the phone or to people I am not familiar with which plays a huge role in me being able to organise my own care."

Does the care you receive consider all aspects of who you are—your physical, psychological and sociological needs?

"No, it does not—now I am older, specialists do not seem to understand my needs, and how my physical needs affect me emotionally and socially. For example, when I went to a local GP about a recent shoulder dislocation, it was evident that

he didn't seem to understand how I was feeling and how much pain I was in, and the effect this was having on my emotional health and daily living. He was very dismissive of me.

I feel the care I receive now is nothing in comparison to when I was younger. It's like all of a sudden, I'm an adult so I no longer matter, and that's how it makes me feel, but thankfully my mum and dad are my advocates, and make sure all my health and emotional health needs are met. If I were not to have this support, I would be very lost in a system I don't understand or feel supported by."

We can see from Georgia's formulation (Table 4.1) how the above accounts have impacted her mental wellbeing throughout her journey. This emphasises the importance of building better joined up working between services.

FAMILY AND OTHER RELATIONSHIPS

We can see from Georgia's formulation how important her family are for her and her health needs. This is reflected in research and current health policy (Department of Health and Social Care, 2023; NICE, 2021). As Luttik (2020) states, people *"need their family and their social relationships in order to stay healthy, to recover from illness or to live with chronic conditions"*. However, the effects that physical health difficulties have upon the family dynamic and other relationships impact significantly. There are feelings of fear, helplessness and frustrations from family members which can conflict with the drive and determination to help the person to "live their best life". The feelings of uncertainty of the child's prognosis and health and lifestyle outcomes alongside feelings of guilt from genetic disorders can have the potential to significantly impact upon the parents' own mental health (Chi et al., 2024). Though the involvement of family is important, this also has the potential to add to the emotional burden of the person emphasising feelings of guilt and resentment of being a "burden" due to the amount of dependency that the person has on family members.

Families often report feelings of frustration and guilt and support is often needed to be able to accept these feelings and to give encouragement to air these so that they can be acknowledged and worked through to prevent a projection of these feelings onto the person and vice versa. This is often something that is very difficult for families to do or admit to, which is why it is an important consideration when looking at formulation which includes family members.

When there are siblings in the family the impact on them can also lead to further feelings of guilt as is demonstrated in Georgia's mother's account. This cannot be ignored, and these impacting factors need to be considered and addressed in the formulation of care. It may be that it is appropriate to have a full family approach and involve the sibling(s) in the process so that their role, thoughts, feelings and motivations are also understood.

Georgia's parents have been a positive influence and significantly important in her care. When considering formulating care, it is important that there is an understanding of their thoughts, feelings and motivators. Some of these have been captured here as they have and will continue to play a significant role in her life.

How did it make you feel as parents when you found out about Georgia's health conditions?

Georgia's mother: *"Initially both myself and Gav were very scared. We were always on edge, waiting for Georgia to become unwell again, we had open access to the children's ward, which was ongoing, due to how suddenly Georgia would become unwell. The diagnosis and illness affected my mental health. I became easily tearful, scared to be on my own with her and needed a lot of family support.*

However, it was Gav who found strength and determination to make sure Georgia achieved her milestones. He took her to all surgeries, he is the one who supported me in attending health appointments and admissions. He was the one who said she would come through this and over time I started to feel that there was hope for Georgia, and that's when my fight began.

Initially, we were worried about the long-term impact on Georgia's future— what would the world mean for her, how would she cope, would she be accepted/ But given that we had an excellent family and community network, we knew she would achieve all she sets out to do."

What has been the most difficult thing about supporting Georgia's health needs over the years?

Georgia's mother: *"The multiple hospital appointments and admissions, coordination of care and management of multiple symptoms.*

Georgia has required referrals to multiple hospitals over the years. She has been under the care of many different services, such as cardiology, neurology, OT, SALT, Physiotherapy, Orthoptics, Orthopedics to name a few, and this was hard to keep on top of. The most difficult has been having to watch Georgia struggle with the changes to her health, when she was first given a wheelchair, how that took away her independence even more, and watching her struggle with her emotions and experience pain like she has. All we ever wanted to do was to take it all away from her.

It was difficult to manage multiple appointments, attend school/EHCP (early help care planning) meeting and work full time.

Watching Georgia struggle with her mental health and experience multiple emotions in one day, due to pain and frustration of being different to others, when all she ever wanted was to be the same.

Georgia could flip from being very happy, to becoming tearful, to being angry, as she struggled to manage and understand herself. She never really had a sense of self-belonging to start with.

As she became older, she was able to adapt, she understood her own limitations in regard to her physical health, but she continues to struggle when others treated her differently, excluded her from parties or events, as they thought she wouldn't be able to manage. This was hard to watch as a parent, it was heartbreaking.

When under children's services we did feel well supported, but since transitioning to adult services, this has become much harder. I feel that I must fight for everything. She has quickly become lost in a system that no longer understands her. If Georgia didn't have parents that helped and assisted her in accessing and requesting services, she would have many unmet health needs and she would deteriorate rapidly both physically and emotionally. This again is hard for us as parents. We are trying to promote her independence, we want her to be able to access services, feel heard and understood, but the battle continues, and it feels like there will never be any rest from this."

How has this impacted upon your family lifestyle? (Holidays, activities, work, etc....)

Georgia's mother: *"Through no fault of Georgia, family life has been hard as we have always had to plan our holidays to suit Georgia's needs. For example, we would only book holidays to countries with good health care, that was accessible. We had to plan insurance in advance which was an additional cost to family breaks. Holidays were restricted, our youngest daughter wasn't able to undertake activities that she wanted to do, such as snorkeling, water parks, as Georgia wasn't able to access them. (Sister) would become frustrated, although she did understand as she had learned to adapt to Georgia's needs too.*

There are many activities we liked to do as a family. Me and Gav have always been active and adventurous and this had to stop. No longer did we go off walking or book random breaks. Everything had to be planned to precision—medication, prescriptions, equipment, accessible support at airports. But she's worth it.

For (sister) it was hard, as I would describe her as an active outgoing young lady. She was exposed to some very difficult situations when Georgia fell ill. She was often present when ambulances arrived, both at home and in other countries. This has left (sister) feeling very anxious around health and hospitals, even now and she's 17. She will openly admit that she worries about being ill, as she doesn't want to go through what Georgia did.

Work was very supportive to us. We were thankful we had private health care in the early years, as we both had to take a lot of time off work, and this helped us out financially. Again, we had a very supportive family network, who had a good understanding of Georgia and we relied heavily on them to offer support when we were working."

How has it made you feel when you have seen how much Georgia has struggled? Have you ever been offered any support for you as a family to manage this?

Georgia's mother: *"The main support we have had is that of family and friends, and of course Georgia's long-term pediatrician. We have never accessed any external support, nor were we offered it. I think this was linked to our resilience, and ability to manage, and the wider family support we had. See letter I have included (Fig. 4.2); this gave us strength to carry on"*

"Although we managed, we still struggled, it was hard to watch Georgia struggle, it was hard to see her cry when she was excluded from events, such as parties. It was even harder to watch her in pain, and we felt completely useless and helpless. There were often nights where I would sit and cry, and feel so alone in it all, sometimes I thought is this all life has to offer, what's the point in carrying on, but it was Georgia and her determination that saw me through. It was her amazing personality and resilience that allowed us to carry on, her commitment and drive to succeed in everything she did that shone through. We couldn't be any prouder of the young lady she has become, which is strong, and independent, achieving all she set out to do. Most of all she proved everyone wrong."

Dear Parent/Guardian of Georgia Grainger

It was a delight to see Georgia walk into clinic and look so well.

These are the little rewards that Doctors look forward too, after committing many years of hard work.

You both have done extremely well to get Georgia to where she is. I hope you take this letter as a record of my appreciation for a family that has worked so well with the health care professionals to get the best outcome for their child.

Thankyou once again for your co-operation.

I remain,

Yours sincerely

Fig. 4.2 Letter from Georgia's paediatric doctor to Georgia's parents

How supportive have you found her healthcare services? Now she is in adult services how difficult is it to continue to co-ordinate her care?

"*Early years—pre-adult—fantastic support, continuity of care, excellent care coordination—it felt like people cared, understood. We even received a thank you letter from Georgia's pediatrician thanking us as parents for being her advocate and fighting for her.*

Transition to adult services has been hard, Georgia no longer has one person coordinating her care. Her care now solely relies on me and Gav, and we have to fight for it. She is under multiple services, all of whom no longer have a good insight into her needs, they don't use an MDT approach. Each service treats one condition, they don't come together to explore how one condition impacts on the other and how these impact on Georgia. I've also found that they speak over Georgia, they speak to me, it's as though she's not in the room. They will often say 'what do you think mum?' 'What do you want from this appointment?', I have to encourage professionals to speak with Georgia, and encourage Georgia to do the same. Georgia will say what's the point, they don't understand me? And that's hard to hear. I've found we now have to replay Georgia's story and health needs over and over to professionals.

The one consistency had been her GP, the practice has been our family practice from birth, and they really do get Georgia, they prioritise her appointments, and will make referrals as and when needed. But again, Georgia would never access the GP independently, and relies on me now she is older to support her.

The only service Georgia has accessed independently is Pain Management—she had some Health Psychology Sessions, and the consultant was what I would describe as amazing, He introduced himself to Georgia, he was patient, he understood her and focused on building a relationship with her before undertaking any work. Georgia really valued this, he validated her feelings and it's the first time she has ever said 'he believes me mum.' When I asked her what she meant by this, she said 'he really believes me, he believes I have pain, he understands how it makes me feel'...and she attended all sessions independently. This service proved invaluable to Georgia, and she is able to access this again when and if needed to in the future."

What are your concerns for the future?

"My honest concerns are:

Will Georgia ever live a fully independent life—I would like to think so, but it's so hard to think this far ahead.

Will she ever have a relationship and experience love in a different way...

I think Georgia will always need an element of support both physically and emotionally moving through life and adulthood. She is very vulnerable in terms of strength, again both physically and mentally.

Georgia's physical health will likely deteriorate further when she is older, how will she cope with this?

Without support, Georgia will not have access to the health care she needs."

As a family you have a really supportive and inclusive culture. What do you think helps to keep this relationship like this?—because as we know in other families this is not always the case and the stress can break families.

"I believe it's down to our morals and family dynamics, we have an excellent supportive family in terms of grandparents, mine and Gav's relationship is great, we are always open and honest, and speak openly about our feelings. I also think it comes from our own childhood backgrounds/history. I came from a divorced single parent family who lived in poverty, family is so important to me. Gav comes from a wealthier background with parents who remained together, and he felt safe and secure. Together we complement each other.

It has been stressful, but Gav is the calm side of our relationship, and I am the one who will voice concerns, and together we keep each other grounded."

You have a really open and honest relationship with Georgia about her health, has this always been the case? Why do you feel this is important?

"Yes, it has, we have always spoken to Georgia about her health needs and limitations, as she needed to understand why she felt different to others and why often, she was excluded from events. Georgia would often be in denial about her health and Autism, so we had to be led by her, with what she should and shouldn't know about her health, and we did it gradually over time, so that it felt natural and not overwhelming.

Georgia had the ability to understand what was happening, and although sometimes it was upsetting for her to hear, we would shed tears together, and find a way to move on as a family.

I firmly believe this is why we remain so close now. Georgia's relationship with her dad is lovely to see. She trusts him unconditionally and really looks up to him. He has helped her to grow and shine from a child to a young adult. He has been the rock of our family and we would have been lost without him.

Having an open and transparent relationship has helped us to manage our day-to-day struggles as a family, we are aware of each other's anxieties/feelings and feel able to speak about them openly."

Including family in the process of formulation is important, this may be at every step of the journey or it may only be appropriate at certain times depending upon the person's (Georgia) choice. This is more complex when you are supporting a child, depending on the child's age and capacity. Some of the complexities of this are when a child is having difficulties due to a family dynamic or the parents have a different motivation or agenda. Establishing this is very important and having a family interview (as demonstrated above) would help to gain an idea of the family situation and motivations.

Completing this type of interview also helps from a strengths-based approach to formulation, as the family's strengths are able to be identified, and the supporting structures (such as parents supporting each other and identifying their strengths in certain areas of Georgia's care).

Sometimes families find it difficult to talk openly and freely when everyone is all together for fear of upsetting, and so a flexible approach may be appropriate. However, in Georgia's family's situation the openness and transparency has been something that has been a strength throughout her life and care, and has helped the family accept when someone is struggling stepping in to support each other as needed.

Mental Health Nursing Perspective

From formulating Georgia's experiences, we can now see the protective factors that she has which can now be used to formulate what might be helpful moving forward for her. It is important that how this moves forward is Georgia's choice as she needs to be in charge of her own life. By completing a formulation in this way it can be used to help Georgia in seeing her journey and understand some of the thoughts, feelings and behaviours that she has developed over time and why. It can then also be used to help you work together in developing a pathway of care. For example, it might be that because Georgia has identified that her pain management has been helped by having psychological support, it might be that she would find psychological support helpful for building relationships or confidence building in new situations.

This biopsychosocial formulation is an overview formulation of Georgia's life experiences, and going forward it could be useful to make a more targeted formulation in a specific area such as looking at relationships or pain management when out of the home environment. It is important to remember that formulation is not a static process, it continues to grow and develop and can be used in many different areas in a person's life to help them explore what are the impacting factors on their journey, and help them to see a different pathway using their own strengths, skills and abilities. It can be used to help identify any methods of coping which they may not have realised they have developed, and for some people these may have been helpful in the short term, but not necessarily helpful in the longer term (such as using substances to help with sleep, these may have helped in the short term but over a long term often develop into a dependency and have health implications).

As Georgia's family are so important to her and have been invaluable in her journey, some of their perspectives have been added to the formulation here. This is because they have seen different aspects of Georgia during her journey and it was important to capture this, but also the need to recognise their concerns in terms of the ongoing journey as this may contribute to some of the choices made in the next steps.

GEORGIA'S SUMMARY

"The process of contributing to the book has proved invaluable to me, even though when I first had sight of the draft chapter it made me quite tearful, it has also helped me to feel validated, someone actually wants to hear my voice, and this means a lot to me. I have now graduated from university, graduating with a first-class honors in Early Childhood Studies, an achievement I am very proud of. My long-term goal is to gain Early Years Teacher Status."

SUMMARY

This chapter identifies the importance of recognising the impacts of a person's physical health upon their mental health and vice versa. Neither one can be treated in isolation. For people with chronic health conditions the impacts of this can be lifelong on a person's mental wellbeing. Using the 4Ps biopsychosocial approach to formulation is a useful tool, helping to identify the impact of the biological and sociological areas of a person's life, upon their psychological needs. Combined with seeing how the predisposing, precipitating and perpetuating factors impact upon each other, helps both the practitioner, but more importantly the person to see their journey and gain an understanding of what the impacts of these areas are/have been on them.

The chapter has identified the importance of collaborative working between services and the impact that this has had upon Georgia's care and mental health, including when it was effective and when it was not.

Points for Reflection
1. Consider in your own practice when you have supported someone with both physical and mental health needs. Could using the 4Ps biopsychosocial model have been helpful?
2. How effective has your collaborative working practice been?
3. What impact did collaboration have on the person you were supporting?
4. How could this have been improved?

REFERENCES

Anti-Bullying Alliance. (2016). *Prevalence of bullying.* https://anti-bullyingalliance.org.uk/tools-information/all-about-bullying/prevalence-and-impact-bullying/prevalence-bullying

Asmussen, K., Fischer, F., Drayton, E., & McBride, T. (2020). *Adverse childhood Experiences. What we know, what we don't know, and what should happen next.* Early Intervention Foundation.

Barker P. (1995) *The child and adolescent psychiatry evaluation: basic child psychiatry.* : Blackwell Scientific, Inc.

Bunn, S. (2021). *Health inequalities: Health conditions and interventions.* UK Parliament Publications. https://post.parliament.uk/health-inequalities-health-conditions-and-interventions/

Chi, Z., Devine, R. T., Wolstencroft, J., et al. (2024). Rare neurodevelopmental conditions and parents' mental health – How and when does genetic diagnosis matter? *Orphanet Journal of Rare Diseases, 19,* 70. https://doi.org/10.1186/s13023-024-03076-2

Copeland, E. (2002). *Wellness Recovery Action Plan. A system for monitoring, reducing and eliminating uncomfortable or dangerous physical symptoms and emotional feelings.* file:///C:/Users/peirs/Downloads/WRAPworkbook-adults.pdf

Dahlgren, G., & Whitehead, M. (1991). *Policies and strategies to promote social equity in health.* Institute for Futures Studies.

Department of Health and Social Care. (2023). *Guidance. The NHS Constitution for England.* https://www.gov.uk/government/publications/the-nhs-constitution-for-england/the-nhs-constitution-for-england

Engel, G. L. (1977). The need for a new medical model: A challenge for biomedicine. *Science, 196*(4286), 129–136.

Felitti, V. J., Anda, R. F., Nordenberg, D., Williamson, D. F., Spitz, A. M., Edwards, V., Koss, M. P., & Marks, J. S. (1998). Relationship of childhood abuse and household dysfunction to many of the leading causes of death in adults: The Adverse Childhood Experiences (ACE) Study. *American Journal of Preventive Medicine, 14*(4), 245–258. https://doi.org/10.1016/S0749-3797(98)00017-8

Harris, M., & Fallot, R. (Eds.). (2001). *New directions for mental health services: Using trauma theory to design service systems.* Jossey-Bass.

Hartley, S. (2021). Using team formulation in mental health practice. *Mental Health Practice.* https://doi.org/10.7748/mhp.2021.e1516

Johnstone, L., & Dallos, R. (2014). *Formulation in psychology and psychotherapy. Making sense of people's problems* (2nd ed.). Routledge, Taylor & Francis Group.

Labinjo, T., Serrant, L., Ashmore, R., & Turner, J. (2020). Perceptions, attitudes and cultural understandings of mental health in Nigeria: A scoping review of published literature. *Mental Health, Religion & Culture., 23*(7), 606–624. https://doi.org/10.1080/13674676.2020.1726883

Luttik, M. L. (2020). Family Nursing: The family as the unit of research and care. *European Journal of Cardiovascular Nursing., 19*(8), 660–662. https://doi.org/10.1177/1474515120959877

Macrae, J. (1995). Nightingale's spiritual philosophy and its significance for modern nursing. *The Journal of Nursing Scholarship, 27*(1), 8–10. https://doi.org/10.1111/j.1547-5069.1995.tb00806.x

McCrory, E., and the UK Trauma Council, Anna Freud. (2024). *How the brain adapts to adversity.* Anna Frend. https://www.annafreud.org/get-involved/networks/uk-trauma-council/

National Institute for Care and Health Excellence. (2021). *Babies, children and young people's experience of healthcare.* NICE guideline [NG204] Published: 25 August 2021. https://www.nice.org.uk/guidance/ng204/chapter/Recommendations

National Institute for Health and Care Excellence. (2011). *Common mental health problems: Identification and pathways to care.* Clinical guideline [CG123] Published: 25 May 2011.

National Institute for Health and Care Excellent. (2009). *Depression in adults with a chronic physical health problem: recognition and management.* Clinical guideline [CG91] Published: 28 October 2009.

Naylor, C., Parsonage, M., McDaid, D., Knapp, M., Fossy, M., & Galea, A. (2012). *Long-term conditions and mental health – The cost of co-morbidities.* The King's Fund, & Centre for Mental Health.

NHS England. (2019). *The NHS Long Term Plan.* www.longtermplan.nhs.uk/publication/nhs-long-term-plan

NHS England. (2023). *RightCare physical health and mental illness scenario.* NHS England. https://www.england.nhs.uk/long-read/rightcare-physical-health-and-severe-mental-illness-scenario/

Niel, K., Hunnicutt-Ferguson, K., Reidy, D., Martinez, M., & Zeichner, A. (2007). Relationship of pain tolerance with human aggression. *Psychological Reports, 101,* 141–144. https://doi.org/10.2466/PR0.101.5.141-144

Nursing and Midwifery Council (NMC). (2018). *Future nurse standards.* https://www.nmc.org.uk/globalassets/sitedocuments/standards-of-proficiency/nurses/your-future-nurse.pdf

Office for National Statistics. (2018). *Children's and young people's experiences of loneliness: 2018.* https://www.ons.gov.uk/peoplepopulationandcommunity/wellbeing/articles/childrensandyoungpeoplesexperiencesofloneliness/2018

PsychDB. (2024). *Biopsychosocial model.* https://www.psychdb.com/teaching/biopsychosocial-case-formulation

Public Health England. (2018). Research and analysis. Chapter 5: inequalities in health. Published 11 September 2018. https://www.gov.uk/government/publications/health-profile-for-england-2018/chapter-5-inequalities-in-health

Sampson, E. L., White, N., Lord, K., Leurent, B., Vickerstaff, V., Scott, S., & Jones, L. (2015). Pain, agitation, and behavioural problems in people with dementia admitted to general hospital wards: A longitudinal cohort study. *Pain, 156*(4), 675–683.

Stoll, R. (1979). Guidelines for spiritual assessment. *American Journal of Nursing, 79*(9), 1574–1577.

Sweeney, A., & Taggart, D. (2018). (Mis)understanding trauma-informed approaches in mental health. *Journal of Mental Health., 27*(5), 383–387. https://doi.org/10.1080/09638237.2018.1520973

The Campaign to End Loneliness. (2022). *The facts and statistics.* https://www.campaigntoendloneliness.org/facts-and-statistics

The Office for Health Improvement and Disparities. (2021). *Guidance. Culture, spirituality and religion: Migrant health guide, Advice and guidance on the health needs of migrant patients for healthcare practitioners.* https://www.gov.uk/guidance/culture-spirituality-and-religion

Weerasekera, P. (1993). Formulation: A multiperspective model. *The Canadian Journal of Psychiatry, 38,* 7.

World Health Organisation. (2021). Comprehensive mental Health Action Plan 2013–2030 World Health Organisation. ISBN: 9789240031029.

Formulating Interpersonal Conflict, Relationship Factors and Abuse

Vickie Howard, Amina Adan, and Naomi Marlow

Key Learning Points
- The significance of relationships and attachments in our lives
- Recognising trauma and its impacts in childhood and adulthood
- Applying differing formulation approaches to an autobiographical account which includes experiences of interpersonal conflict, relationship factors and abuse.
- Seeing strengths and hope
- Applying formulation to mental health nursing practice

INTRODUCTION

Relationships and how we navigate through them in our lives can have an overwhelming impact on our wellbeing, behaviours and outlooks. This chapter will examine in particular how detrimental relationships through family members, partners, care givers and trusted others can have a devastating effect on our

V. Howard (✉)
Faculty of Health Sciences, University of Hull, Hull, UK
e-mail: V.Howard@Hull.ac.uk

A. Adan
Tavistock and Portman NHS Trust, London, UK
e-mail: AAdan@Tavi-Port.nhs.uk

N. Marlow
Miami, FL, USA

© The Author(s), under exclusive license to Springer Nature Switzerland AG 2024
V. Howard, L. Alfred (eds.), *Formulation in Mental Health Nursing*,
https://doi.org/10.1007/978-3-031-59956-9_5

development and mental health, taking into account childhood experiences and the lack of opportunity for them to be acknowledged and/or supported. We will begin by reviewing some of the key underpinning and theoretical literature in these areas before moving on to look at an autobiographical account which presents a number of situations around relationships and more specifically abuse, where themes of abuse throughout childhood and adulthood occurred. These will be examined through differing approaches to formulating these experiences in combination with the individual who experienced them. You will hopefully see that this is quite a journey here for all involved in this formulation, which has involved a good deal of reflection. These approaches and what has been learnt will be further considered for what can be taken away and applied to mental health nursing practices and our values as mental health nurses. As you read through this chapter, be aware of any issues which may surface for yourself and write them down if you can. These may be things you may want to revisit, either in relation to your own practice (through clinical restorative/developmental supervision) or through personal support routes.

Childhood Experiences

The impact of adverse childhood experiences has been said to be vastly under considered in the presentations of adult mental distress, with the majority of people using mental health services never being asked about child abuse or neglect (Read et al., 2017). Even though there has been a focus on recognising adverse childhood experiences (ACEs), there is still disparity in just how much these early experiences have been acknowledged, explored further and taken into consideration if an individual presents with severe distress or problems with behaviour in adulthood (Tzouvara et al., 2023). These statements are made with consideration to the assessment and 'treatment' routes for mental health problems in the health services in the UK. The UK referral, assessment and intervention routes may be comparable to other countries in that there are processes around service referral waiting times, times to access assessment/ support and expected discharge indicators. It is probable that all of us may not fit neatly into these systems and that the exploration of childhood experiences and how they may be impacting on our adult wellbeing is not an area for extended exploration in a pressured mental health service. This is not a doom and gloom statement, but rather a chance to reflect on what is written here and question: is this my experience, as a student? A nurse? Another health or social care practitioner? Someone trying to access support? Do we give people the opportunity to express themselves and talk about childhood experiences and consider if anything has impacted on them which still leaves a significant consequence, confusion or distress....? We will leave this with you to think about..... and move on to some specifics of distress....

Trauma in Childhood

What may be considered as trauma in childhood is an important starting point, when considering what may be impacting on a child right through to adulthood and being mindful of presenting problems or distress and possible childhood connections to adulthood distress. Trauma in childhood may span a vast array of individual experiences. The National Child Traumatic Stress Network (NCTSN, 2023) advise that children who have been in situations where they feared for their lives, believed that they would be injured, witnessed violence or tragically lost a loved one may show signs of child traumatic stress. They identify the following experiences as traumatic stress:

- Physical, sexual, or psychological abuse and neglect (including trafficking)
- Natural and technological disasters or terrorism
- Family or community violence
- Sudden or violent loss of a loved one
- Substance use disorder (personal or familial)
- Refugee and war experiences (including torture)
- Serious accidents or life-threatening illness
- Military family-related stressors (e.g. deployment, parental loss or injury)

The National Child Traumatic Stress Network (NCTSN, 2023) summarise that without treatment, repeated childhood exposure to traumatic events can affect the brain and nervous system and increase health-risk behaviours (e.g. smoking, eating disorders, substance use, and high-risk activities). Research shows that child trauma survivors are more likely to have long-term health problems (e.g. diabetes and heart disease) or to die at an earlier age. Traumatic stress can also lead to increased use of health and mental health services and increased involvement with the child welfare and juvenile justice systems. Adult survivors of traumatic events may also have difficulty in establishing fulfilling relationships and maintaining employment.

The Indicative Trauma Impact Manual (Taylor & Shrive, 2023, p. 164) highlights that trauma can interfere with a person's ability to develop healthy attachments with others which in turn can lead to various attachment issues. This is an important area to consider with regard to how attachments may have been formed, both secure and negative, and/or how they have been interrupted throughout a person's life. As Taylor and Shrive (2023) continue, discerning specific attachment experiences with family or partners may yield specific instances which have been detrimental through betrayal, gaslighting, abuse, harm and neglect.

DOMESTIC VIOLENCE

Domestic violence, which may also be represented by other language terms such as domestic abuse or intimate partner violence—is a phenomenon which spans across all ages, genders, races and sexual orientations (Alejo, 2014). It is indicated that more women (1 in 4) than men (1 in 6) experience domestic violence (Department of Health, 2017).

Key discernments exist between male domestic violence against women and female domestic violence against men. This comprises of women's experience of higher rates of victimisation and serious harm (Walby & Towers, 2017; Women's Aid, 2023) and additionally women are more likely to be killed by a male/male (ex)partner within domestic violence (Office for National Statistics (ONS), 2023). Higher levels of fear and a higher prevalence of experiencing coercive and controlling behaviours have also been connected to women's experiences of domestic violence (Dobash & Dobash, 2004; Myhill, 2015). However, it has been identified that women often do not report domestic violence to the police (HMIC, 2014). This results in the contextual features of the abuse remaining unclear which enables ongoing disparity in the understanding of the gendered nature of domestic violence.

Domestic violence has historically been framed in physical injury manifestations which did not support those in the helping professions to also assess and be aware of the more invisible signs of abuse and injury (Shipway, 2004). Although it can be argued that this is still in its infancy, contemporary health and social care services now recognise more hidden forms of abuse including psychological and emotional abuse. Coercive control, which is characterised by coercive or controlling behaviour within an intimate or family relationship is an offence under Section 76 Serious Crime Act 2015 (Crown Prosecution Service, 2023). Such behaviour often includes economic, emotional and psychological abuse. This can also include threats and may include physical and sexual violence and abuse (Home Office, April 2022). A related form of abuse includes narcissistic abuse, though this is largely unheard of throughout society and within the helping professions. Narcissistic abuse is carried out by an individual deemed to have severe narcissistic traits including a lack of conscience and a primary need to bolster their own self-esteem. Like coercive control, it can include financial, emotional and psychological, physical and sexual abuse. It has been proposed that narcissistic abuse can be distinguished from other forms of abuse by the perpetrator's use of deception towards the victim to execute dominance and control, and that the deception in itself should be recognised as a form of abuse (Milstead, 2018). There is currently no legislation to protect victim-survivors from individuals inflicting this form of abuse.

THE IMPACT OF RELATIONSHIP DISTURBANCES IN ADULTHOOD

The issues highlighted in the preceding sections identify key points which can help us reflect on the possible individual factors and life experiences which may be detrimentally impacting on a person's relationships and wellbeing. The below autobiographical account by 'Naomi' (pseudonym) portrays both childhood and adult experiences and begins to build a picture of how these may have impacted on current problematic areas. However, within this account it is evident that Naomi holds many strengths. As you read through this write down what you consider Naomi's strengths are and the areas you would want to discuss further with her.

NAOMI'S AUTOBIOGRAPHICAL ACCOUNTS

Here is my childhood: Born oldest of 2 children in a 2 parent middle class household. Significant hypothyroidism and eczema from birth. My dad had a massive MI when I was 7. He almost died and it was found later the MI was secondary to polycythemia vera. My mom lost her voice for a couple years due to the stress. No memorable abuse until after my little brother who is 3 years younger than I am was born. He had life threatening asthma and my parents were preoccupied keeping my brother breathing. Dad was a functional alcoholic and coped by taking us to his mother's sister's house more and more frequently. This is where I was molested by her second husband, starting at about 6 years old to 9. My molester told me to tell no one because no one would believe me. I tried to just avoid the old creep, but when he retired, he had all day to drive around and stalk me—try to touch me. At 9, I told my mom who dragged my dad into the mix. I was given a week's break from visiting my molester. My dad wanted to control the narrative that the molestation happened only once. The stalking continued. I can remember trying to leave school and get in the woods to walk home as fast as possible. It was also difficult to ride my bike around town, because I felt I just didn't belong or deserve to be part of life. I gained weight after the molestation. Maybe partly due to terrible and lacking thyroid control. School was a 10 year nightmare where I was verbally and physically attacked and bullied. I did have some close friends. It was very comforting to make art or play instruments. Functionally I was fat and socially odd. When the abuse started with the molester, my little child mind wanted someone to save me from the crime but no one came. The one thing I thought was *"There must be something wrong with me."* Because no one came, because I wasn't loveable.

My maternal grandmother was so kind to me. Mom was so supportive of anything I wanted to do especially art and traveling playing violin. I had some friends but was an independent loner. I rarely followed rules which made my father so angry with me. He would tell people what a horrible child I was. I remember in my late teens asking my dad why he didn't report the crime that happened to me. His response was "What would your poor Aunt Charlotte think if she found out, it would hurt her terribly." This was the molester's wife. Things were never the same after with my dad. I understood in his eyes I was not good enough to be loveable or even protected from a criminal. I never even pointed out how his response made him look like a shit father.

When I tell parts of my story, I wonder how I lived through it... The lesson to take from my story is that childhood neglect and abuse causes lifelong issues when you weren't taught that you are the most important person. My health is utter shit from the years of believing I was unlovable. I spent decades looking for men to make me feel loved and safe. It is a separate nightmare story. During this time, I worked obsessively and had my own house and enviable savings. It is all gone now thanks to being sick and the NPD (Narcissistic Personality Disorder) wasband. Therapy has been hit or miss. Chump Lady (a blog on leaving abusive relationships) saved my life 8 years ago. I have always had weekly therapy. Learning to sit calmly with myself is the best therapy and learning about CPTSD (complex post-traumatic stress disorder). Richard Granton is a huge factor in my survival to date. He understood and articulated the phenomena of NPD abuse. Before this, I felt like an alien on this earthly planet.

(Shows a photograph) This is my camp on 3 acres with an outhouse. I can't stay in this house, but I plan escapes for 3 season camping along the rugged northern coast of Maine. This is where I have wanted to be for decades… I dug deep and paid cash, which is a miracle after my divorce and being penniless and homeless. I need land clearing, but have the money. It is hard to hire help in a town of less than 600. But it will be done some day. I will fix the a- frame so it is a nice shelter.

I am thinking of how I am going to put together my adult distress. I was wondering if you had any interest in me discussing the last couple of years in relation to Covid 19, political, and global issues in relation to my health. I guess I should preface all of this by saying I was a quiet liberal and after having several of my own businesses and owning a home, I quietly shifted my political leanings to conservative because it offered me opportunity to be more free and less regulated in my charitable work. I am conservative but not loud or pushy. I enjoy a rich diversity of political beliefs.

I was vaccine injured, early 1970s, as a child and told no more jabs. I had 2 of the Hep B shots back in 1993 after brow beating by my employer. My eczema, asthma, thyroid issues were distressingly uncontrollable. I complained to my docs re being sick and relating it to the mandatory jabs for work. I was told I was crazy and suffered in pain for the better part of a year and lost my dream job. After almost a year of suffering a nightmare autoimmune flare I ended up in the emergency room with a thyroid storm—myxedema. I believe this was the starting point for the pile on of new and more complicated autoimmune issues. No one believed me… but I resolved no more shots to excite my immune system, because my body historically got the immune response wrong and I need things like my lungs, liver, pancreas, etc.

I had been treated with HCQ for my autoimmune issues starting in 2019. It was helping a little… With the advent of Covid 19 and orange man Trump having taken HCQ, I was abruptly DC'd and put on a new and very expensive Xeljanz by Pfeizer. Because HCQ was too controversial, even though it worked. Anyway, I took the Xeljanz and was advised early spring 2021 that there had been reports of clotting issues with Xeljanz and suggested a switch to Humira, I already had a failed trial and bad reaction to that. I stayed the course with Xeljanz because my skin on my hands was perfect and I was getting joint relief.

I am almost back to normal now, I am so grateful it wasn't worse, but I HAD A STROKE on August 21. I had a STROKE not just a TIA. I have 2 small areas of brain damage in watershed areas. They found a left internal branch carotid artery thrombosis with a 60–75% occlusion. While in the hospital, I found 5 new black box warnings for Xeljanz in regards to thrombosis, MI, and CVA with all kinds of attorneys looking for injured patients for a class action law suit. You know my rheumatologist who initially warned me told me it couldn't possibly have been the drug, same with the stroke team… cover for Pfizer much?

I believe there are nice people in this world, but the falling away of all long-term friendships because I simply voted for the wrong president or happen to hold fiscally conservative beliefs was disheartening. I feel quite alone and disoriented. My family is toxic and disheartening in and of itself. So I feel isolated in my home and have no friends to visit or call.

As you can imagine even before my stroke, I spent lots of time in medical settings for appointments. Since my stroke, it has become so clear to me that in Massachusetts, there is some kind of social cast system based on political orientation, vaccine status and race (I happen to be Hawaiian) and when I insist on having my demographics recorded correctly, I am laughed at half of the time and told my race doesn't count. Uh, OK, white man occupied my ancestors' land and brought diseases that killed all but 20% of native Hawaiians. The US took our sovereignty, things went so horribly for the native Hawaiians that President Bill Clinton actually apologized. But I digress…

Stroke related hospital visits… the first question is always did you get your Covid 19 vaccine. When I was having my stroke, the triage nurse asked if I got my vaccine and I told her I was vaccine injured as a child and then again in the 90s which became a battle that my excuse did not count as a medical exception and she wanted me to agree to the vaccine right then and there. I didn't and boy was she angry… I was sent to a room right in front of the nurses' station. There was a mental health patient just tiring himself out, an extremely hypertensive octogenarian female, a 30 something girl who stepped on a nail and me… The woman who just had right side weakness and lost the use of my hand before coming to the hospital. IV nurse came and asked if I had the Covid 19 shot, attending asked, the EKG tech asked, vitals girl asked… everyone asked me. Was my 'no' answer the reason they left me for 3 hours lying there in a ghost town ER as punishment before they brought me to the CT scan and I was still asked vaccine status. After the CT, I heard all kinds of activity at the desk with my attending doc. As a result of the delay, I couldn't get the clot buster and was put on heparin and sent to a teaching hospital in town and when I arrived again everyone's first question, "Did you get the vaccine?"

I have never judged people based on their race, political ideals, sexual orientation, medical status, etc. I just cannot imagine discriminating like this. I am flabbergasted by the way I see people behave. My trust with the medical establishment here is almost gone. I am not anti-science or anti vax but why the hell have I become a second class citizen with my freedoms further eroded every day because I am selfish, stupid, anti-science. I was injured as a child it caused life changing long-term autoimmune flares. Why can't I have an exception? I am a human too… I get to hear how horrible I am from the President and his administration. I hear main stream media mocking me and saying people like me don't deserve medical treatments or meds.

I am not suicidal. Honestly, all the previous abuse I suffered helped me see this for what it is… And yes, I believe people were getting sick and dying. I see this as a very narcissistic global organization working their hardest to injure, terrorize and separate people from each other. I have felt alone, friendless, hurt, angry, but I have learned to cope with this before and I can cope with being alone going forward. But it truly pains me that there are others who are being hurt and dying because of the way things are… that makes me the most distressed. Just like at the end of my marriage, my wasband was going to widow and widower dances lying that I was dead. Most likely he was trying to kill me then, but I felt bad for the widows he was deceiving long before I felt bad for myself.

Politics and Covid have not improved my life one bit… I am so emotionally labile and all over the place with the next upsetting subject of the day. When I am done pondering the world the way it is, I dissociate and go mentally dead for a while. Here in the Midwest, we had tornadoes before Christmas. I decided to work or volunteer with our emergency management or Red Cross to get away from my family and help others worse off than me. I was asked if I had the vax and then when I gave my answer, I was told they didn't want people like me.

I am just trying my best to cope. I want to cultivate a better relationship with God, the world around me and my fellow man. I want to live free and in peace. It is my goal to find a peaceful like-minded community. Oh, and when Covid blows over I intend to write about my experience as a regular consumer in the medical industry and include some parallels to the way things were in the 80's working with AIDS patients during the AIDS epidemic. It sure is eerily similar…. I hope this wasn't too triggering for you. I also believe there are still good people in the medical industry, but we sure are in weird times.

Reactions to Autobiography

Within formulation approaches (as within a range of therapeutic interactions and approaches), it is important to consider our own reactions to others' experiences and stories. Our (Vickie and Amina's) reflections and reactions are outlined below and reiterated by Taylor (2010, p. 101) when she talks of 'feelings and in-tuneness'—

> "In-tuneness is clearing away the debris of rationality, to face up to, and embrace, the rawness of emotions, which when expressed unblock the streams of human reactivity and cause our life energies to flow a little easier. In-tuneness is an essence of being human, by relating to another human through sensitive expressions of feeling."

Vickie

I found this a very moving account of experiences. What struck me was the alone and isolated child without an advocate or 'rescuer' from the child abuse. When I was reading the childhood account, I wanted to leap in and protect the child from the child sexual abuse and to also acknowledge and tell the child I believed her, not change the narrative as she had experienced from her father. As well as the abuse, was the neglect by her father and denial with no response to protect which I found equally disturbing and upsetting. The societal impacts on the dominant discourses around Covid 19 were also very striking and health professionals' attitudes and responses. As a health professional this stuck a very deep chord and I was emotionally saddened around the lack of compassion and lack of trying to understand Naomi's experiences. Naomi's thoughtful and critical inquiry and working towards and establishing her own space, property and land was inspiring to me.

Amina

Reading Naomi's account of childhood abuse invoked an intense sense of anxiety and vulnerability in me. Her explicit description left me feeling overwhelmed. A sense of aloneness crept over me as I moved through each line of her account. I wondered about the impact of her trauma as she reflected on the defensive strategies she mobilized to keep herself safe and psychologically intact. I was left with thoughts of the damaging legacy of chronic child abuse on Naomi's sense of self and felt a sense of alienation. Her longing for a land of her own struck me as hopeful.

Naomi

Reading my account back I feel it is like looking in on someone else.

Formulation Perspectives

In order to begin looking at current distress, issues and problematic areas, we can begin piecing together what has happened to Naomi throughout her life. There are a number of approaches which can be considered for this and we will use some of these approaches to look at Naomi's experiences and how these may have impacted on her. Naomi herself will reflect on these and offer her views and what may or may not resonate with her and what may have resulted in viewing her thoughts and experiences through alternative lenses.

A CBT Approach to Formulation

Dudley and Kuyken (2014) suggest a framework for CBT formulation that supports an individual to link their experiences to the cognitive model. This is

Table 5.1 Applying the 5Ps of CBT formulation to Naomi's experiences

The 5Ps	Naomi's experiences—Vickie and Amina's observations	Naomi's views
Presenting issues What are the person's presenting emotions, thoughts, behaviours and difficulties?	Isolation, lack of social contacts, disconnect. Complexities of physical health. Lack of trust in professionals' judgements and advice.	I often feel people don't take the time to try to understand.
Precipitating factors What factors triggered the person's current difficulties and presenting issues?	Childhood trauma was a precipitating factor, however Naomi identifies judgements of health professionals as a triggering factor in her suspicion and lack of trust in professionals which can often occur.	My childhood included some disturbing experiences. I think sometimes the way I am treated takes me back there.
Perpetuating factors What are the external and internal factors which continue the person's current difficulties?	There is a sense of feeling judged by health professionals which does not provide any validation to Naomi. A continuation of not feeling understood which leads to feeling low in mood and occasionally avoiding social situations or appointments as a means of self-protection.	Feeling disconnected and not understood.
Predisposing factors What factors increased the person's vulnerability to their current problems?	Childhood experiences of abuse affecting trust and disrupted attachments with key care givers. Being reminded by the attitudes and behaviours of healthcare professionals, her experiences are not acknowledged and validated. Ongoing anxieties about the actions of her ex-husband and his threatening behaviour. Naomi associates her choice of partner with her disrupted attachments in childhood and being taken in by an initial charming person who later showed himself to be untrustworthy, dishonest and abusive.	Trauma experiences.
Protective factors What are the person's strengths and resilience that help them maintain their health?	Naomi's ability to reflect and make sense of her experiences. Creativity, arts interest and connection with nature. Finding a safe place to live and feel nurtured.	Relationship with God. Finding safe and nurturing places.

referred to as the 5Ps of CBT formulation and includes exploration of the person's presenting issues, precipitating factors, perpetuating factors, predisposing factors and protective factors. We are using this framework to apply to Naomi's experiences which is represented in Table 5.1. A 5Ps approach to formulation is often used during assessment to establish a contextual picture of a person's presenting problem(s). Throughout the formulation, a consideration of the therapeutic relationship is key and discussing aspects of the 5Ps may give a good opportunity for developing trust and showing empathy to develop collaborative understanding.

CBT can also be used to break down a problem and a 5 areas formulation can be used for this. Naomi's 5 areas formulation below in Fig. 5.1 is based on a model developed by Padesky and Mooney (1990). The diagram shows how all the 4 areas below the situation (or 'environment' in Padesky and Mooney's description) connect with each other and the situation. A maintenance of the problematic situation may be in effect. The thinking is that changing

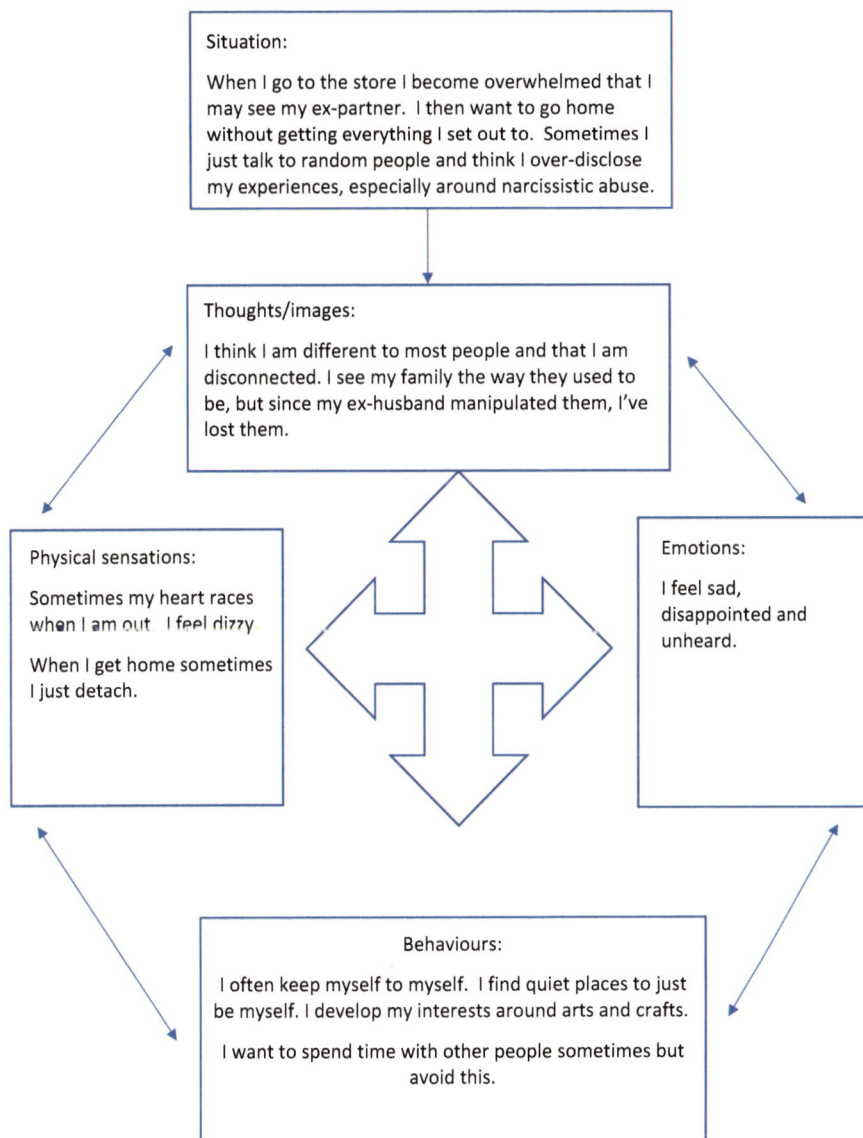

Situation:

When I go to the store I become overwhelmed that I may see my ex-partner. I then want to go home without getting everything I set out to. Sometimes I just talk to random people and think I over-disclose my experiences, especially around narcissistic abuse.

Thoughts/images:

I think I am different to most people and that I am disconnected. I see my family the way they used to be, but since my ex-husband manipulated them, I've lost them.

Physical sensations:

Sometimes my heart races when I am out. I feel dizzy

When I get home sometimes I just detach.

Emotions:

I feel sad, disappointed and unheard.

Behaviours:

I often keep myself to myself. I find quiet places to just be myself. I develop my interests around arts and crafts.

I want to spend time with other people sometimes but avoid this.

Fig. 5.1 Naomi's 5 areas formulation

something in one of the areas may have a positive effect on one of the other areas and therapist and client can examine all the areas and begin identifying action points from the client's perspective of what they may want to change.

A Psychodynamic Approach to Formulation

There are several approaches to case formulation in psychodynamic assessment and Treatment (Eells, 2010). Psychodynamic formulation serves as a tool for constructing hypotheses about a person's inner world, encompassing their thoughts, emotions and behaviours. It places a particular emphasis on the influence of unconscious processes and how they unfold over the course of their developmental history. This invaluable tool allows us to construct hypotheses that explore the depths of a person's inner world—capturing their thoughts, emotions and behaviours in a comprehensive tapestry. It's essential to acknowledge that a person's growth is sculpted by a unique interplay between their genetic makeup and the environment that surrounds them. Psychodynamic formulations are not rigid, fixed explanations but rather flexible hypotheses that can be adjusted and refined as new insights emerge (Cabaniss et al., 2013).

What sets psychodynamic formulations apart from other types of case formulations, such as CBT formulations, is their specific focus on delving into the impact of unconscious thoughts and feelings on an individual's difficulties. By exploring these hidden realms of the mind, psychodynamic formulations shed light on underlying factors that contribute to challenges individuals may face. This approach underscores the significance of raising individuals' awareness of their unconscious processes, as it serves as a key technique in psychodynamic interventions. Through this process, individuals gain valuable insights into themselves, paving the way for personal growth and transformation (Trimboli & Farr, 2000).

Mental health professionals oriented towards psychodynamics place particular importance on understanding a patient's childhood, as it is crucial in comprehending the development of unconscious thoughts and feelings. This knowledge can be applied in various ways during treatment, including helping patients recognise how their current behaviour is influenced by past experiences, supporting the development of capacities that were not fully formed during childhood, and addressing impaired functioning resulting from acute or chronic issues.

Naomi's autobiographical accounts reveal several unconscious dynamics that have shaped her psychological functioning. One notable unconscious dynamic is repression, as she describes repressing the memories of the childhood molestation and the ongoing stalking by her perpetrator (Fonagy & Sandler, 1997). Repression is the defence mechanism that blocks or pushes distressing or traumatic memories, thoughts, or desires out of conscious awareness to prevent them from causing overwhelming anxiety (Freud, 1915). This repression is likely a defence mechanism employed to protect herself from overwhelming feelings of fear, shame and powerlessness.

Another unconscious dynamic evident in Naomi's narrative is identification with the aggressor. She internalises the message that there must be something wrong with her because no one came to save her from the crime. This identification serves as a way to maintain a sense of control and self-worth in the face of trauma. It also explains her subsequent self-perception as unlovable and her pattern of seeking validation and love from others, particularly men (Kernberg, 1984).

Naomi's object relations, or her internalised representations of relationships with significant others, have been profoundly impacted by her early experiences (Fairbairn, 1952; Klein, 1946). Her mother appears as a supportive figure who encouraged her interests in art and music, providing a sense of security and nurturance. Conversely, her father's response to the molestation and his prioritisation of protecting his sister-in-law over Naomi shattered her trust in him and undermined her sense of worthiness for protection and love (Fairbairn, 1952). This betrayal and neglect from a significant parental figure significantly impacted her object relations and self-perception.

These early object relations experiences influence Naomi's current relationships, as she struggles to form and maintain long-term friendships and feels isolated and disoriented. She may have difficulty trusting others fully, fearing abandonment and rejection, given her past experiences of not being protected or believed.

In response to the overwhelming trauma and subsequent emotional distress, Naomi employs various defence mechanisms to cope with her experiences. Repression, as mentioned earlier, enables her to keep traumatic memories out of conscious awareness. This defence mechanism shields her from the full impact of the trauma but also inhibits her from fully processing and integrating those experiences into her conscious mind (Freud, 1915).

Another defence mechanism that emerges in Naomi's narrative is displacement. She redirects her anger and frustration towards the medical establishment and society at large, feeling marginalised and discriminated against due to her political beliefs, vaccine injury and racial background. This displacement helps her manage her intense emotions by externalising them onto others, allowing her to maintain a semblance of control and protect her self-image (Freud, 1914).

Given Naomi's history of trauma and neglect, transference and countertransference dynamics are likely to emerge in therapeutic relationships. In transference, Naomi may unconsciously transfer unresolved feelings, attitudes and expectations onto her therapist. For example, she may project onto mental health practitioners the need for protection, validation, and a sense of being heard and believed. Countertransference refers to the therapist's emotional reactions and subjective experiences in response to the client's transference. Naomi's history of trauma and complex emotional struggles may evoke strong countertransference reactions in workers, such as feelings of compassion, empathy, and a strong desire to help and protect her (Klein, 1946).

It is important to acknowledge that a psychodynamic formulation is not a definitive explanation but rather a tool to enhance treatment methods and understanding of patients. Similar to hypotheses, psychodynamic formulations are formulated, tested and revised. The process of formulating psychodynamically does not conclude upon generating a hypothesis; rather, it continues throughout the course of treatment. The formulation represents an evolving understanding of the patient and their development. The clinician and patient continuously learn about new patterns and history, leading to the generation of new hypotheses and the refinement of understanding.

Formulating psychodynamically ultimately involves a continuous mode of thinking for clinicians. Although it is beneficial to document psychodynamic formulations to consolidate ideas and practice skills, not all formulations need to be written down. Psychodynamic thinking occurs during interactions with patients, when considering their needs, and determining appropriate interventions. The goal is for clinicians to integrate the skills learned in psychodynamic formulation into their daily practice with all patients.

Trauma-Informed Perspectives

Looking at Naomi's experiences and asking 'what has happened to you?' rather than 'what is wrong with you?' immediately helps us to focus in again on Naomi's 'story.' This approach to inquiry in attempting to understand an individual's distress has been outlined in The Power Threat Meaning Framework-PTMF (Boyle & Johnstone, 2020). A key point of the PTMF is that narratives and stories can replace psychiatric diagnosis and that a damaging effect of psychiatric diagnosis can obscure personal meaning (Boyle & Johnstone, 2020, p. 32). As outlined in the introductory chapters to this book, the PTMF encourages understanding of a person's distress or problematic experiences in the context of relationships, social situations and the expectations of how we are expected to respond and live. Naomi's account of her experiences particularly links to what the PTMF has to say about the importance of recognising social and political influences on individuals' experiences. For example, Naomi describes how she feels overwhelmingly judged regarding her outlook on obtaining or not obtaining the Covid vaccination and how this has caused some distress and disharmony. Boyle and Johnstone (2020, p. 31) highlight the importance of the roots of what we may call mental health problems, which may be based on judgements about what we ought to think and feel. These are often based on values rather than objective medical criteria and feeling that we may not be living up to or are unable to conform to these expectations may cause great distress. In Naomi's case, even though she has the courage of her convictions, processing and dealing with the reactions and judgements of others still causes distress and barriers to accessing compassionate support and physical healthcare. In addition, the cultural and societal issues Naomi highlights with regard to the non-recognition of her Hawaiian heritage are important factors and in her story contribute to an experience of not being heard.

A Strengths Approach

The Strengths Model (Rapp, 1997) highlights the importance of recognising and drawing upon an individual's strengths as a means of growth and recovery and connecting with the community and environment to access an oasis of resources (Rapp & Goscha, 2006). The relationship of the 'worker' in the strengths framework is also highlighted as essential and they are viewed as a travelling companion to assist the distressed person to see opportunities, their talents and skills and attain their life goals. The helping relationship sees the worker having genuine investment and motivation in respecting an individual's autonomy and self-determination, whilst supporting life goals an individual may express or have. When applying the principles of a strengths approach to exploring Naomi's distress, challenges and situation there are a number of areas for discussion. Naomi clearly articulates what she has as internal and external resources. She talks about the importance of her environment and has secured her own land and is working on a home environment on the land. Through her internal strength and determination, she owns this goal and continues to develop it.

The PTMF also identifies the recognition of a person's strengths as an important area and uses the language of 'power resources.' What stands out here for us is Naomi's…'*skills and abilities, such as intelligence, resourcefulness, determination and particular talents*' (Boyle & Johnstone, 2020, p. 35). Naomi also expresses sourcing particular crucial information at particular times of distress to support her with processing distress and working out her experiences (via Chumplady online and Richard Grant to identify aspects and experiences of narcissistic abuse). Another approach to working with and recognising people's strengths can be identified in the field of psychology where the term 'positive psychology' is used.

Naomi's Views on These Formulations

It does help to look at what I have been through in my life, but to also get some recognition of this. I realise though I have worked through a lot of things and am a strong person and also empathetic towards others. I actually feel quite proud of myself…I am who I am.

Towards an Integrated and Extended Application of Formulation in Mental Health Nursing

There are a number of areas from these illustrated formulation examples which we can reflect upon and question how as mental health nurses or mental health professionals we can be mindful of the main learning points, and how this resonates in our practice and indicated therapeutic interventions and care plans. We are going to discuss these further below:

Attachments, Relationships and Abuse

Listening to Naomi's accounts of betrayals and/or abuse within familial and intimate relationships highlights the trauma experiences she has endured both as a child and adult. Earlier in this chapter, ACEs were outlined as an important consideration in identifying previous experiences influencing current mental distress and problematic areas. John Read, Professor in Clinical Psychology also advocates for the term *adverse life events* and explains he feels it is more inclusive of adverse experiences which may not meet the criteria for trauma but can be just as debilitating (Read & Winn, 2023).

In particular, Naomi portrayed her experiences of invisibility when she was subjected to childhood sexual abuse and this was not recognised and then minimised by her father. Naomi's description of both trauma and adverse life events and the effects this had on her development and outlook leading to adulthood and adult relationships led to Naomi's following statements.

> *"When I tell parts of my story, I wonder how I lived through it… The lesson to take from my story is that childhood neglect and abuse causes lifelong issues when you weren't taught that you are the most important person. My health is utter shit from the years of believing I was unlovable. I spent decades looking for men to make me feel loved and safe. It is a separate nightmare story."*

In formulation practice, it is advised that formulation is an ongoing process and that gaps in information and knowledge may be apparent and information and discussion will be developed and revisited (Johnstone, 2014). What Naomi has discussed, but not in a lot of detail to this point—is that her ex-husband is a current source of concern and distress. She has described him having NPD (narcissistic personality disorder) and as a result she has identified she has experienced narcissistic abuse (or as expressed by Naomi; NPD abuse). This is a key consideration when thinking about the current problem areas and distress Naomi is experiencing and how this may span across and inter-connect with past/other areas of her life. Although 'narcissistic abuse' is a term not commonly understood or used within society or within health and social care, it is emerging from survivor networks and research as an essential area of abuse which requires further recognition because of the devastating impact it can have on victim-survivors and those around them. As authors of this chapter, we are aware of and study narcissistic abuse, undertaking scholarship and research aiming to build understanding of the experiences of the victim-survivor and the integral drivers of the narcissistic individual (see Howard, 2019 and Howard & Adan, 2022).

Within further discussion, Naomi has identified;

"I don't have children. My husband is still dragging me to court long after the divorce to wear me down and destroy me financially. He even reported my art to social security disability, stating I was defrauding the system and could work. He has just about killed me… I had a vanco pic line at discard and I believe he was drugging me to kill me."

Within nursing practice, concepts may come to us which we have little knowledge on or which are new to us. Narcissistic abuse may be an example of this to some mental health nurses or mental health professionals reading this. Examining how an individual's reported experiences of narcissistic abuse interrelate to others' reported experiences of narcissistic abuse may help us formulate their experiences and understand some of the mechanisms of abuse used towards the victim-survivor (e.g. the abuser eroding an individual's sense of self to maintain control over them in order to meet their own self-esteem needs). An article Vickie produced in 2019 (Howard, 2019) particularly highlights the importance of mental health nurses' understanding of the presentations and patterns involved within narcissistic abuse because often mental health nurses may be the first mental health practitioners to provide assessment to a distressed individual and so they are in a prime position to identify signs of narcissistic abuse. Although narcissistic abuse is complex in its presentation because it can be insidious and the victim-survivor's accounts of their abuse may seem far-fetched and sometimes unbelievable, this again is a flag for further investigation with regard to both risk and safety issues which need consideration for the victim-survivor and what they are reporting they have experienced.

Using Formulation to Understand, Develop the Therapeutic Relationship and Identify Support Approaches

We can summarise that the benefits of using formulation approaches centre on 1) developing an understanding of an individual's presenting problems and strengths. 2) That the process of formulation has the potential to build upon the therapeutic alliance and therapeutic relationship between helper and person seeking support and 3) The information gained through the formulation process can underpin and inform directions in establishing therapeutic interventions or approaches which may support an individual to move forward in areas of their life or address problematic experiences. The seminal work of Peplau (1952, 1988) emphasises the therapeutic relationship in the context of interpersonal relations theory suggesting that interactions that occur between nurse and patient have qualitative impact on outcomes for the patient. The following excerpt taken from Peplau's (1952, 1988, p. xii) highly influential publication *Interpersonal Relations in Nursing: A Conceptual Frame of Reference for Psychodynamic Nursing* foregrounds contemporary approaches identified in collaborative formulation practices which emphasise the importance of the therapeutic alliance:

Nurses are also in a position to identify and study degrees of skill that people use in struggling with presenting difficulties and to develop with patients the kinds of new experiences that are needed for such skill improvement. Assistance in the identification of problematic situations, appreciation and liberation of positive forces in patient personalities are functions of the nurse. As each nurse helps a patient to identify problematic elements in his current situation and to discover and understand something about what is happening to him during his illness, she both expands her own insights and helps the patient to grow.

Peplau (1965, p. 20) ascertained that *"Every human being needs to explain to himself what is happening to him and why."* Throughout the development of her theories within nursing she identified within 'psychiatric nursing' that interventions with individual patients centred on *nurse-patient relationships.* However, the language she used changed, moving to *one-to-one relationships,* then *counselling* and ultimately *psychotherapy* (Werner O'Toole & Rouslin Welt, 1994). However, there was a disparity and discomfort in using the term *nurse psychotherapists* and other terms were used which were deemed less threatening and more acceptable (Werner O'Toole & Rouslin Welt, 1994). This is an interesting historical point to consider with regard to how we as mental health nurses explain our skills and background when building the therapeutic relationship with an individual and also within explaining our skills regarding formulation.

And so following the collaborative formulation process leads to a question of—now what?

At this junction there may be a range of options available for helper and individual to explore. These may involve considerations involving the preference of the person being supported and may also be underpinned by what the helping professional and the service criteria entails and offers. Examples of therapeutic interventions may come under the umbrella of psychologically informed interventions and a range of 'talking therapies' and if considering the biopsychosocial approach (Engel, 1977) how interventions targeting the biological, psychological and social factors involved in a formulation may indicate what may help an individual with problem areas.

However, when considering mental health nursing and therapeutic interactions throughout the formulation process, there are a number of perspectives which may help us stand back and consider for ourselves what may be important. One of these areas is the 'therapeutic use of self.' Val Wosket (2017, p. 11) ascertains; *"Use of self involves the operationalisation of personal characteristics so that they impact on the client in such a way as to become potentially significant determinants of the therapeutic process."*

Considering how we use aspects of ourselves and the notion of spending time with a person in distress—what this time means and the value of it—are often at the centre of the realities of situations we find ourselves in as mental health nurses. Tony McSherry (2018, p. 234) adds to this consideration:

"In this way too, 'theorising' about mental health nursing may be missing something uniquely individual about the therapeutic person. For example, think about sitting with someone during the night who has tried to strangle themselves, about trying to 'be with' that person. The therapeutic aspect in these hours and moments may have nothing to do with medication, diagnosis or psychological formulation and everything to do with the person of the mental health nurse and how she or he has come to be."

Using Formulation as a Component of Mental Health Nursing and Multidisciplinary Practice

The above identifications of the benefits of formulation and the foundation it may serve in identifying future supportive interventions integrate well with therapeutic mental health nursing. For example, in the process of assessment, intervention and review as part of the care planning process, it can be recognised how formulation can fit in to this nursing process. However, in consideration of formulation, there are additional factors we can question and explore for the mental health nurse's role:

Where Does Formulation Fit in for the Mental Health Nurse's Role in Exploring Safety?

When reading back through the formulation viewpoints and approaches presented, there may be questions which may have popped into your head with regard to your own practice. One such question may be concerned with safety, risk assessment and risk management and where this may fit in within the formulation approaches outlined. In practice, risk assessment is usually completed as a specific (electronic) document within an initial screening assessment, examples of such risk assessments being FACE (Imosphere, 2023) and HR-20 (Douglas et al., 2014). In addition, it is expected areas of risk will be checked and re-evaluated during contacts and appointments. Upon discussing the 'presenting problem' in the 5Ps formulation, there may also be discussion on problematic areas and/or behaviours which progress on to risk assessment discussion to establish areas which may be impacting on the individual's safety or that of others. These discussions may also indicate safeguarding issues which will require action in accordance with the Trust or service policy and escalation procedures.

SUMMARISING KEY AREAS OF THIS CHAPTER

This chapter has outlined an autobiographical account in Naomi's own words about her childhood and adult experiences relating to relationships, attachments and abuse. Differing ways of looking at Naomi's experiences through formulation have been presented and discussed with a consideration to components which can be further considered in mental health nursing practice. The main messages for us as chapter authors centre around the importance of really trying to understand and listen to a person we are working with, whilst showing respect, compassion and a genuine sense of empathy whilst examining our own internal processes and thoughts. Additionally, Naomi has voiced that this process and talking through her experiences has made her consider what she has been through in her life, giving her a sense of strength and herself.

Points for Reflection

1. **Interpersonal Conflict and Personal Growth** Reflect on how personal experiences with conflict and abuse have shaped your understanding of trauma and resilience. How can these insights inform your approach to mental healthcare?

2. **Childhood Experiences and Adult Mental Health** Consider the impact of ACEs on adult relationships and mental health. How does this knowledge influence your perspective on therapeutic interventions?

3. **Formulation Approaches in Practice** Explore the significance of formulation in mental health nursing. How can integrating these approaches enhance care and support recovery?

4. **Empathy and Therapeutic Relationships** Reflect on the role of empathy and compassion in healing. How do these qualities affect the outcome of therapy for trauma survivors?

5. **Professional Growth through Personal Reflection** Think about how your personal background influences your professional practice in mental health nursing. How can continuous reflection and learning improve care for individuals experiencing trauma?

References

Alejo, K. (2014). Long-Term Physical and Mental Health Effects of Domestic Violence. *Themis: Research Journal of Justice Studies and Forensic. Science, 2*(5) https://doi.org/10.31979/THEMIS.2014.0205; https://scholarworks.sjsu.edu/themis/vol2/iss1/5

Boyle, M., & Johnstone, L. (2020). *The power threat meaning framework*. PCCS.

Cabaniss, D. L., Cherry, S., Douglas, C. J., & Graver, R. A. (2013). *Psychodynamic formulation*. Wiley-Blackwell.

Crown Prosecution Service (CPS). (2023, April 24). *Controlling or coercive behaviour in an intimate or family relationship*. Retrieved from CPS: https://www.cps.gov.uk/legal-guidance/controlling-or-coercive-behaviour-intimate-or-family-relationship

Department of Health. (2017). *Responding to domestic abuse: A resource for health professionals*. Department of Health.

Dobash, R., & Dobash, R. (2004). Women's violence to men in intimate relationships: Working on a Puzzle. *British Journal of Criminology, 44*(3), 324–349.

Douglas, K. S., Blanchard, A., Guy, L., Reeves, K., & Weir, J. (2014). *HCR-20 violence risk assessment scheme: Overview and annotated bibliography. HCR-20 Violence Risk Assessment White Paper Series, #1*. Mental Health, Law, and Policy Institute, Simon Fraser University.

Dudley, R., & Kuyken, W. (2014). Case Formulation in cognitive behavioural therapy: A principle driven approach. In L. Johnstone & R. Dallos (Eds.), *Formulation in psychology and psychotherapy: Making sense of people's problems* (2nd ed., pp. 18–44). Routledge.

Eells, T. (2010). *Handbook of psychotherapy case formulation*. Guilford.

Engel, G. L. (1977). The need for a new medical model: A challenge for biomedicine. *Science, 196*(4286), 129–36. https://doi.org/10.1126/science.847460

Fairbairn, W. R. (1952). *Psychoanalytic studies of the personality*. Routledge.

Fonagy, P., & Sandler, C. (1997). *Recovered memories of abuse true or false?* https://doi.org/10.4324/9780429479427

Freud, S. (1914). *The psychopathology of everyday life. Standard Edition* (Vol. 6).

Freud, S. (1915). Repression. *The Standard Edition of the Complete Psychological Works of Sigmund Freud., 14*, 141–158.

HMIC. (2014). *Everyone's business: Improving the police response to domestic abuse*. HMIC.

Home Office. (2022, April). *Controlling or coercive behaviour statutory guidance framework*. Home Office.

Howard, V. (2019). Recognising narcissistic abuse and the implications for mental health nursing practice. *Issues in Mental Health Nursing, 40*(8), 644–654. https://doi.org/10.1080/01612840.2019.1590485

Howard, V., & Adan, A. (2022). "The end justifies the memes": A feminist relational discourse analysis of the role of macro memes in facilitating supportive discussions for victim-survivors of narcissistic abuse. *Cyberpsychology: Journal of Psychosocial Research on Cyberspace, 16(4), Article 10*. https://doi.org/10.5817/CP2022-4-10

Imosphere. (2023). FACE Assessment Toolsets. https://imosphere.com/care-and-support-tools/face-toolsets/

Johnstone, L. (2014). Controversies and debates about formulation. In L. Johnstone & R. Dallos (Eds.), *Formulation in psychology and psychotherapy* (pp. 260–289). Routledge.

Kernberg, O. (1984). *Severe personality disorders: Psychotherapeutic strategies*. Yale University Press.

Klein, M. (1946). Notes on some schizoid mechanisms. *The International Journal of Psychoanalysis*, 99–110.

McSherry, T. (2018). Mental health nursing as therapy. In J. Bull, J. Gadsby, & S. Williams (Eds.), *Critical mental health nursing: Observations from the inside* (pp. 226–245). PCCS Books.

Milstead, K. (2018). *Defining narcissistic abuse: The case for deception as abuse*. Retrieved from PsychCentral: https://psychcentral.com/lib/defining-narcissistic-abuse-the-case-for-deception-as-abuse#1

Myhill, A. (2015). Measuring coercive control: What can we learn from national population surveys? *Violence Against Women, 21*(3), 355–375.

NCTSN. (2023). *About child trauma*. Retrieved from NCTSN: https://www.nctsn.org/what-is-child-trauma/about-child-trauma

Office for National Statistics (ONS). (2023, July 15). *Domestic abuse victim character-istics, England and Wales: year ending March 2022.* Retrieved 2023, from Office for National Statistics: https://www.ons.gov.uk/peoplepopulationandcommunity/crimeandjustice/articles/domesticabusevictimcharacteristicsenglandandwales/yeare ndingmarch2022#domestic-homicide

Padesky, C., & Mooney, K. (1990). Clinical tip: Presenting the cognitive model to clients. *International Cognitive Therapy Newsletter,* 13–14.

Peplau, H. (1952). *Interpersonal relations in nursing.* G.P Putnam's Sons.

Peplau, H. (1965, February). Interpersonal relationships in nursing Paper presented at Council on Hospital Services Institute, District of Columbia-Delaware Hospital Association, Washington DC.

Peplau, H. (1988). *Interpersonal relations in nursing.* The Macmillan Press.

Rapp, C. (1997). *The strengths model: Case management with people suffering from severe and persistent mental illness.* Oxford University Press.

Rapp, C. A., & Goscha, R. J. (2006). *The strengths model: Case management with people with psychiatric disabilities* (2nd ed.). Oxford University Press.

Read, J., Harper, D., Tucker, I., & Kennedy, A. (2017). Do adult mental health services identify child abuse and neglect? A systematic review. *International Journal of Mental Health Nursing, 27*(1). https://doi.org/10.1111/inm.12369

Read, W., & Winn, D. (2023). Lack of insight: The story of psychiatry. *Human Givens Journal, 30*(1), 30–31.

Shipway, L. (2004). *Domestic violence: A handbook for healthcare professionals.* Taylor & Francis.

Taylor, B. (2010). *Reflective practice for healthcare professionals.* Open University Press.

Taylor, J., & Shrive, J. (2023). *Indicative trauma impact manual: A non-diagnostic, trauma-informed guide to emotion, thought, and behaviour* (1st ed.). VictimFocus.

Trimboli, F., & Farr, K. L. (2000). A psychodynamic guide for essential treatment planning. *Psychoanalytic Psychology, 17*(2), 336–359. https://doi.org/10.1037/0736-9735.17.2.336

Tzouvara, V., Kupdere, P., Wilson, K., Matthews, L., Simpson, A., & Foye, U. (2023). Adverse childhood experiences, mental health, and social functioning: A scoping review of the literature. *Child Abuse & Neglect, 139.* https://doi.org/10.1016/j.chiabu.2023.106092

Walby, S., & Towers, J. (2017). Measuring violence to end violence: Mainstreaming gender. *Journal of Gender-Based Violence, 1*(1), 11–31.

Werner O'Toole, A., & Rouslin Welt, S. (1994). *Hildegard E. Peplau, selected works.* The Macmillan Press LTD.

Women's Aid. (2023). *Domestic abuse is a gendered crime.* https://www.womensaid.org.uk/: https://www.womensaid.org.uk/information-support/what-is-domestic-abuse/domestic-abuse-is-a-gendered-crime/

Wosket, V. (2017). *The therapeutic use of self: Counselling practice, research and supervision.* Routledge.

CHAPTER 6

Formulation Considerations for Individuals Experiencing Emotional Distress and Substance Use

Lolita Alfred and Roselyne Masamha

Key Learning Points
- Understanding substance use, co-occurring emotional distress and associated difficulties
- Exploring different theoretical lenses and how these can underpin formulation
- Exploring religion and context as important areas for consideration
- Trauma informed and culturally sensitive approaches to care
- Longitudinal CBT Formulation situated within the 'APIE' nursing process
- Considerations for the role of mental health nurses in formulation

Introduction

The following chapter explores substance use and co-occurring emotional distress (often recognised as 'dual diagnosis' in psychiatric and mental health settings). The chapter outlines a fictitious case study example that portrays an individual who is struggling with their mental health, using cannabis and

L. Alfred (✉)
City, University of London, London, UK
e-mail: Lolita.Alfred@city.ac.uk

R. Masamha
Engaged Consultancy, Hull, UK

© The Author(s), under exclusive license to Springer Nature Switzerland AG 2024
V. Howard, L. Alfred (eds.), *Formulation in Mental Health Nursing*,
https://doi.org/10.1007/978-3-031-59956-9_6

alcohol as coping mechanisms. An example will be provided of how formulation might be approached in a mental health nursing context—situating formulation within the nursing process. The use of substances and the thresholds that constitute a disorder is an area fraught with challenges relating to definitions, use of terminology, conceptualisations, and debates around substance use as a health issue versus it being an issue of personal choice and responsibility. All of this is situated within an arguably fractured policy context made up of distinct, overlapping and sometimes contradictory directions and guidance. When substance use co-occurs with various states of emotional or psychological distress, the complexities are further compounded. The current chapter briefly examines this complex context, as it contributes to shaping approaches to intervention, and help-seeking for individuals who are struggling with substance use and co-occurring emotional distress. For this chapter, the definition of substance use as '*the recurrent use of alcohol [or] drugs that leads to clinically and functionally significant impairment*' by Earnshaw (2020) will be adopted. The chapter will also refer predominantly to the term 'emotional distress' which is a non-pathologising term to describe a state of emotional suffering or an individual's struggle with their mental health. We acknowledge that in mainstream psychiatry (or diagnostic language) emotional distress would encompass what is understood as mental illness or diagnoses of mental health conditions such as depression, psychosis or bi-polar disorder—to name a few.

POLICY, GUIDANCE AND PUBLIC HEALTH LANDSCAPE

The World Health Organisation (WHO) International Classification of Diseases and the American Psychiatric Association (APA) Diagnostic and Statistical Manual of Mental Disorders provide diagnostic criteria for substance use disorders and mental health conditions. At a global level, several policies and guidance documents address substance use and mental health individually, and as co-occurring health conditions. Some examples worth reading are the World Mental Health Report (WHO, 2022) aimed at transforming environments, attitudes, actions and approaches for promoting and protecting mental health, and providing care and treatment for those that need this; and the Special Initiative for Mental Health: Universal Health Coverage for Mental Health (WHO, 2019) which aims to achieve equitable access to mental health services for mental, neurological and substance use disorders. For substance use, a helpful document is The International Standards for the Treatment of Drug Use Disorders (WHO and UNODC, 2020) which focusses on developing and expanding evidence-based, effective and ethical treatment for drug use disorders, with principles for establishing treatment services and provision of interventions. It is worth noting that for substance use, there are also laws and regulations such as the Drugs Misuse Act (1971) which makes provisions for harmful or dangerous drugs (such as cocaine, heroin) and provides classifications (Class A, Class B and Class C) according to level of harm and enables penalties to be applied for possession or distribution (Pycroft, 2010). However, some substances such as alcohol are excluded from the classification system, despite it being a major contributor to avoidable mortality, morbidity and a wider range of social problems such as crime, violence and poor parenting (Obot & Room, 2005; Department of Health [DH], 2009); and despite its proven impact on 14 out of 17 of the health-related United Nations Sustainable Development Goals[1] (SDGs) which aim to provide a more equitable and sustainable future for all people (Bakke, 2018). There are however other laws and regulations for alcohol, such as those around drink-driving which enable penalties to be issued for those convicted of driving while under the influence of alcohol. At a country level, there are also strategies for drugs and alcohol that serve as national guidance for the approach to public health level and individual level service provision, assessment and treatment. It is not within the scope of this chapter to comprehensively explore all the regulations, policies and guidance documents however the context will be important to bear in mind while reading the chapter and exploring the factors that may be impacting on the individual at the centre of the case study.

Other important contextual aspects to consider are the debates on whether the use of substances constitutes an illness or a lifestyle choice; and the complexities that come with managing substance use as a criminal justice matter, a health issue or both. Approaches to intervention are often reactionary—applied at the point of crisis, for example Hall (1997) highlights that in some cases of substance-related offending, there can be court imposed treatment orders for the individual with a view to this contributing to reducing the risk of re-offending. However, more preventative approaches, and holistic analyses of substance use which recognise and account for the wider circumstances from which substance use emerges are recommended, for example, through considering Marmot's 'causes of the causes', an approach which emphasises the need for a 'deep dive' into wider contributory factors, in order to move away from one-dimensional approaches that position the individual as wholly responsible for their health conditions. Accounting for these wider socio-economic factors, educational exposure and family circumstances are crucial because these factors are also cited as contributing to increased trauma and high levels of stress, leading to mental health deterioration which in turn heightens the risk for substance use. Substance use prevalence, attitudes, and norms vary across groups, settings and cultures. This will be explored in more detail through the formulation and discussed with regard to supporting Tatenda, who we introduce below.

---

[1] SDGs are a collection of 17 interlinked global goals developed by the United Nations General Assembly in 2015. The goals are—No Poverty; Zero Hunger; Good Health & Wellbeing; Quality Education; Gender Equality; Clean Water and Sanitation; Affordable & Clean Energy; Decent Work & Economic Growth; Industry Innovation & Infrastructure; Reduced Inequalities; Sustainable Cities & Communities; Responsible Consumption and Production, Climate Action; Life Below Water; Life On Land; Peace, Justice, and Strong Institutions; Partnerships for the Goals.

CASE STUDY—TATENDA

Tatenda is 36 years old, and she lives with her family (husband and a 9-year-old son) in London. She is of Black African ethnicity, born in the small town of Gokwe in Zimbabwe. She attended a missionary-led primary school followed by another missionary-led boarding high school from the age of 13–16 years. Tatenda left high school without any formal qualifications and after holding a few temporary jobs, she left Zimbabwe at 19 years and moved to London where she lived with a friend for a while. She describes life in London as 'cold and hard' because she was in a new country, different to what she was accustomed to culturally. She also said she felt isolated and lonely because she only knew one or two people, which contrasted with the sense of family she had when she was in Zimbabwe with a large extended family and a wide social circle. Living in London was also very expensive, she soon turned to prostitution to make ends meet. Tatenda feels a sense of shame about this. She met her husband while on the job and describes meeting him as the day that her life changed for the better. Her husband is of White British ethnicity.

From birth until the age of 8 years old, Tatenda's father spent a lot of time away from home as he was in the army. Tatenda lost her mother when she was just 11 years old. Her mother died while in childbirth and the baby also died a few weeks later, a double loss for Tatenda of mother and sibling. Tatenda thinks there was something suspicious about her mother's death, believing her paternal grandmother had killed her mother using witchcraft because she wanted her son to marry another woman. Tatenda's mother was never fully accepted by her husband's family, partly because she was Christian, and the husband and his family were Muslim. Tatenda's mother often experienced verbal and physical violence in the home—most of which Tatenda and her siblings witnessed. Tatenda's father often justified the beatings as a way for him to discipline his wife and assert authority. When Tatenda's mother passed away, Tatenda's father shifted his violence and aggression towards her and her siblings, and she vividly remembers feeling like he used what she referred to as 'military style punishments'.. One time, she decided to fight him back. Tatenda described her father as a violent, and angry man who drank too much alcohol and did not seem like he cared for her even while her mother was alive. Her father abandoned her after the death of her mother, and he refused to pay for her school fees because he said she was a disrespectful, disobedient, and badly behaved child, citing a high interest in boys and promiscuity. Tatenda told her maternal aunt who lived in a different city what was happening, and she stepped in to help pay for her education, moved her to a boarding school and Tatenda would live with her during the school holidays. Tatenda's aunt is Christian and whenever Tatenda went to her home for the holidays, they would go to church every Sunday and her aunt would always pray for her. Tatenda has some fond memories of this time in her life, and the sense of belonging she felt after such a turbulent start to her life.

Tatenda has been recently admitted to an acute mental health ward for assessment as an informal patient, with suspected substance induced psychosis. Her husband was concerned about her as she had not slept for 72 hours, and she had been consuming high amounts of alcohol and cannabis over the past few months, and more recently had been taking energy drinks to stay awake while studying for her final exams for the Marketing Degree she was pursuing. She says the degree was a crucial part of getting a promotion at work. Her husband says she has been talking about her family 'sacrificing her' because they are jealous of her. He says she has been talking about her work colleagues, describing them as evil and whenever she walks into the office, she feels hot and sweaty, and knots in her stomach and says this is because of her colleagues' evil deeds. Tatenda was angry with her husband for suggesting she be admitted to the ward citing disruption to her focus on completing her exams. Having always had pursuing education emphasised, Tatenda felt her husband was getting in the way of her achieving this goal. She also disagrees with the diagnosis she has been given and keeps saying 'I am not crazy'. On the ward, Tatenda expresses low mood, and being overwhelmed by everything; compounded by feelings of pressure to be a good wife, have a good job, have a good education, be a good mother—of which she feels she can never live up to. She recognises and acknowledges their wealth privilege, however, can't help but feel a sense of lack of satisfaction with her life, questioning whether she is deserving of this. Tatenda describes her husband as a very loving man, even though he has on several occasions been physically abusive towards her. She mentions fighting back only occasionally. More recently she has been thinking about her spirituality and she wonders if going to church will help get her life back on track

Considerations for Tatenda's Formulation as a Key Part of the Nursing Process

As identified in the book introduction (Chap. 1), 'Formulation' is usually seen as practice led by Psychologists. Doctors/Psychiatrists also lead on Case Formulation (Goldberg & Murray, 2002). In the example below, we illustrate how mental health nurses could integrate formulation into their day-to-day practice. As a large mental health professional group, who are more likely to spend the most time in contact with individuals who are experiencing distress (e.g. 24-hr care settings), there is scope for developing the mental health nurses role in formulation. There are concerns, at least in the United Kingdom (UK), that the unique aspects that set mental health nursing apart from any other field of nursing are being diminished by the slow move towards generic nurse training (Buescher & McGugan, 2022; Warrender et al., 2024). The opportunity for developing skills in formulation is important for strengthening the unique mental health nursing professional identity, while also ensuring mental health nurses have an additional skillset they can use to help those experiencing emotional distress. As Tatenda has been admitted to an acute mental health ward, the following provides an example of how mental health nurses can contribute towards formulation, as part of the nursing process. The Nursing Process, structured through the stages of; 'Assess, Plan, Implement & Evaluate' (APIE) was developed by Yura and Walsh in 1967, to progress towards a more systematic and evidence-based nursing profession and move away from the historical ritualistic and intuition-based practice (Barrett et al., 2019). APIE is therefore a core part of nursing practice in the UK and it is embedded within the Nursing and Midwifery Council Future Nurse Standards of Proficiency for Nurses (NMC, 2018). The role and expectations of nurses aligned with APIE are clearly articulated in the following platforms

- *Platform 3 Assessing Needs and Planning Care: Registered nurses priori-tise the needs of people when assessing and reviewing their mental, physical, cognitive, behavioural, social, and spiritual needs. They use information obtained during assessments to identify the priorities and requirements for person centred and evidence-based nursing interventions and support. They work in partnership with people to develop person centred care plans that consider their circumstances, characteristics and preferences.*
- *Platform 4 Providing and Evaluating Care: Registered nurses take the lead in providing evidence based compassionate and safe nursing interven-tions. They ensure that care they provide, and delegate is person centred and of a consistently high standard. They support people of all ages in a range of care settings. They work in partnership with people, families and carers to evaluate whether care is effective, and the goals of care have been met in line with their wishes, preferences and desired outcomes.* (NMC, 2018, pp. 13–18)

Figure 6.1 outlines APIE and Fig. 6.2 incorporates an additional stage showing that formulation can be situated between the Assess & Plan stages of the nursing process.

Fig. 6.1   Assess, Plan, Implement, Evaluate (APIE) nursing process

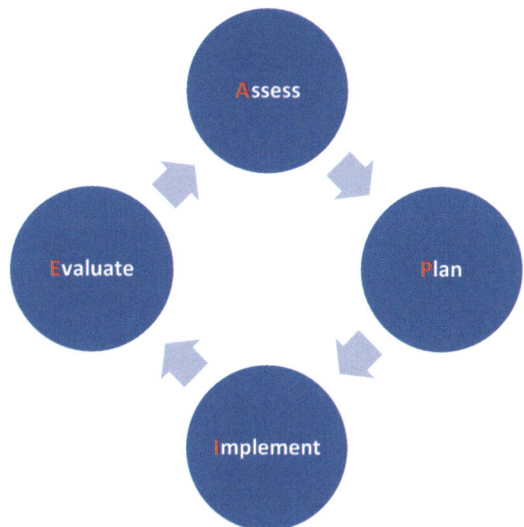

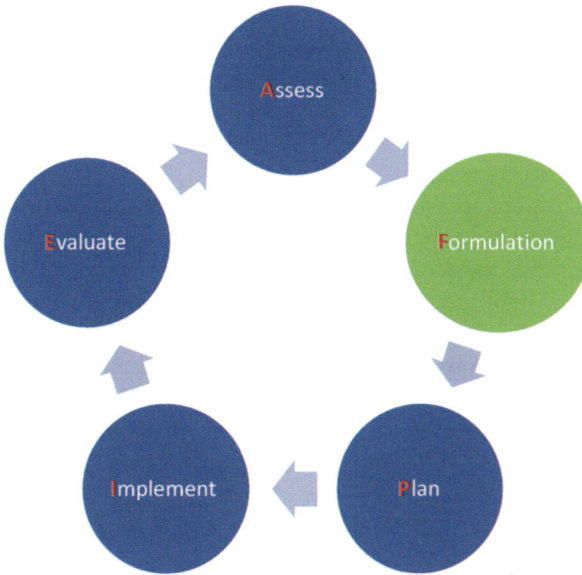

Fig. 6.2 Situating formulation within the APIE nursing process

Assess

To undertake formulation, there needs to be a comprehensive assessment. Mental health nurses already engage in continuous assessment within the clinical settings that they work in. The information gathered at assessment includes data on an individual, their circumstances, health needs, usual routines and the ways they have been managing any health problems (Barrett et al., 2019). This process of assessment would be undertaken collaboratively with Tatenda. Establishing baselines would also be important to give an indication of current areas of need but also to establish any areas of strength and what Tatenda is able to do independently. Baselines also become important when measuring the impact or effect of any interventions implemented and the extent to which these have supported Tatenda's recovery. Tatenda's assessment would also include, with her consent, physical observations, Urine Drug Screening (UDS), blood and other tests such as electrocardiogram. Assessment would also entail outlining Tatenda's coping strategies and gathering information about the ways in which she is currently managing her mental health and substance use. The case study indicates that Tatenda has been struggling with her mental health, and using alcohol and cannabis as coping strategies, but assessment would need to delve a little deeper, going beyond the surface-level presentation in order to understand factors contributing to and maintaining her substance use and experience of emotional distress.

During assessment, an understanding of the individual, their circumstances and the environments that might have contributed to their difficulties, starts to develop. The information gathered at assessment can also contribute to decisions made within the multidisciplinary team (MDT), and to planning care. Assessment should be comprehensive encompassing different areas of physical and mental health, current mental state, family and social history, cultural considerations, and drug or alcohol use (Foster et al., 2020). There are a variety of tools that can aid assessment—for example, the Mental State Examination (MSE), which is used to establish an individual's mental state (Assadi, 2020). The MSE would guide a mental health nurse to establish the nature and content of Tatenda's thoughts, and the level of distress associated with these. At assessment, it is established that Tatenda has been struggling with thoughts of colleagues being evil and meaning her harm, and her family sacrificing her. Assessing Tatenda's insight as part of the MSE would also be important, however this part can often present with a challenge if the mental health nurse establishes Tatenda has lack of insight, while Tatenda views herself as 'not crazy', the practitioner will need to manage this perspective with skill and sensitivity.

Assessing and monitoring risk would be a crucial part of assessment, especially for individuals struggling with use of substances such as alcohol because unmanaged withdrawal symptoms may lead to death. There would be a requirement to develop and implement a risk management plan as documented in the National Institute for Health and Care Excellence (NICE) guidance [CG120] (2011) relating to coexisting mental illness and substance misuse management. Risk assessment is often guided by hospital policy—and at the nursing level involves a formulation approach. Whether mental health nurses recognise this as 'formulation' or not is an area that requires further exploration in research and clinical practice. For example, the '4Ps of Risk Assessment' offer a framework to undertake risk assessment with consistency and transparency (Kaya et al., 2019). This would entail risk 'formulation', even if the term is not explicitly used. Literature identifies that patients are often not involved as collaborators in risk and safety assessments (Coffey et al., 2017), therefore it would be important for Tatenda to be included as a collaborator in her risk formulation.

Thorough and systematic history taking would explore when Tatenda's use of alcohol and cannabis started, the circumstances around that, the changes in frequency of use (as well as current level of use) and what might have influenced or contributed to the different levels or frequency of use. The assessment would also explore any actual or potential impact her substance use may be having on her health. There are assessment tools that can aid this part of the assessment—for example, the Alcohol Use Disorders Identification Test (AUDIT) would give an indication of the level of alcohol consumption and any potential dependence that could be investigated further. Area to be aware of when asking questions around drug and alcohol use is the terminology that is used. For example, in the UK, 'units' are used as an objective measure of alcohol consumed, and identification of the different levels of risk associated with units of alcohol consumed (Department of Health [DH], 2016). Units are calculated through multiplying the volume of alcohol consumed by the percentage strength of alcohol then dividing the result by 1000. The conversation around Tatenda's use of alcohol would also consider that there is variation in how individuals view heavy consumption (Harkins et al., 2010). There are differences in how the public refers to amounts consumed, and these differences also occur across countries—for example, the United States uses 'standard drinks' as a measure whereas the UK uses 'units'.

A conversation around Tatenda's cannabis and alcohol use would additionally need to consider wider factors that may influence the extent to which Tatenda feels able to talk about her substance use. For example, potential fear of implications on employment if she divulges any struggle with alcohol use, and the illegality of cannabis (in the UK) may instil a fear of being open about its use. Tatenda is also a parent, there are additional considerations such as potential fear she may have about the ramifications of admitting to a drug or alcohol problem which may trigger involvement of social services regarding her nine-year-old son. Likewise with her mental health, it would be important to have a sense of when Tatenda began thinking and feeling like her family was sacrificing her or that her work colleagues are evil. This history is important as it can give a sense of whether there are any patterns or links that can be made particularly between substance use and the thoughts she has been having, or if there are other factors contributing to her emotional distress. The history is important for establishing if similar struggles had occurred for Tatenda previously, coping mechanisms adopted and the extent to which these had helped (or not). One aspect to recognise with Tatenda is migration which has implications for the access to any previous clinical records prior to her move to the UK. An important part of assessment would therefore involve gathering information from Tatenda herself and her family, other healthcare providers like family doctor/general practitioner (GP) about her life and health prior to moving to London.

Central to the process of assessment is the therapeutic nurse-patient relationship. Building trust and instilling confidence that Tatenda will receive non-judgemental support would be important given the 'double stigma' that mental ill health and substance use carry. Furthermore, building trust would ensure Tatenda feels safe to seek and receive support from services. There is a comprehensive body of literature that explores stigma which is experienced due to public perceptions (public stigma) and stigma which is self-imposed (self-stigma), and this literature indicates that stigma consistently impacts on help-seeking. Language used is essential for beginning to break down some of the stigma, and there is a helpful language guide that was produced by the Institute of Alcohol Studies (IAS) (2023) that mental health nurses and other professionals can refer to. Bearing in mind that assessment can be affected by several factors such as social and cultural background, physical state (tiredness, stress), emotional state (e.g. motivation, perception of information and events, knowledge base) (Barrett et al., 2019), some considerations for Tatenda may include discussing her perspective on how she is feeling, and exploring how she is framing her experiences through the lens of the environment and culture she grew up with.

Formulation

Formulation involves taking information gathered at assessment, making sense of it using bio-psycho-social theory, and then collaboratively planning care that is informed by the formulation. The central values of formulation are compassion, person centredness, collaboration and trauma informed. These values will be illustrated in Tatenda's formulation and consequent plan of care. Mental health nursing education involves introduction to, and an exploration of a variety of theories, frameworks and research aimed at developing an understanding about emotional wellbeing and human distress—and all this is central to formulation. There is no universally agreed definition of formulation however the following provides a good overview of what it is, and in this chapter, we will draw on elements of all these four definitions

> *Formulation draws on psychological theory and research to provide a framework for describing a client's problems or needs, how it developed and how it is being maintained.* (British Psychological Society [BPS], 2011)
>
> *Formulation is a provisional explanation or hypothesis of how individuals come to present with a certain disorder or circumstance at a particular time.* (Weerasekera, 1996, p. 4 cited in Johnstone & Dallos, 2006, p. 4)
>
> *Biopsychosocial formulation is a way of understanding a patient as more than a diagnostic label, by combining biological, psychological, and social factors to understand a patient, and uses this to guide both treatment and prognosis.* (Engel, 1977; Borrell-Carrió et al., 2004)
>
> *Formulation is a clinical opinion, weighing up the pros and cons of conflicting evidence, which leads to a diagnostic choice.* (Goldberg & Murray, 2002, p. 96)

The main purpose of formulation is to hypothesise how Tatenda's psychological, interpersonal and behavioural struggles are caused and maintained, doing so by using underpinning theories. It is also important to note that formulation is not diagnosis—rather it is about making sense of an individual's experiences and emotional distress. Formulation helps to provide a stronger basis on which to recommend treatment and interventions. It is never complete—this is in recognition that peoples' lives can change from day to day, and a formulation will continue to evolve reflecting any changes happening for the individual. McClelland (2014) outlines that formulation needs to reflect a complex picture where the ambivalences and inconsistencies of inner thoughts and feelings are not simply individually driven, or inherent faults of the person needing to be 'fixed', but part of a social world which is shaped by contradictory and conflicting expectations. With that in mind, let us explore how a mental health nurse might consider the choice of formulation approach.

Choice of Formulation Approach

The decision regarding which formulation approach to use is thought to be influenced by the practitioners' style. However, this can also be done collaboratively between the mental health nurse and Tatenda. Earlier chapters have explored the different approaches such as Psychodynamic Formulation and Cognitive Behaviour Therapy (CBT) Formulation. For Tatenda's formulation, a Classic Longitudinal CBT Formulation might be a useful starting point because Tatenda is expressing distressing thoughts that are of a paranoid nature, to the extent that these have impacted on her home and work life. CBT theory suggests that mental illness can be caused by distorted or irrational thinking patterns and negative behaviours (Taylor & Shrive, 2023). The Longitudinal CBT Formulation can enable connections to be made between Tatenda's thoughts, her feelings, how she responds (in terms of behaviour) and the bodily sensations she has. Longitudinal CBT Formulation also considers early life experiences, schemas and conditional beliefs which will be important to understand for Tatenda particularly because we have information about her childhood experience of several traumas that may have impacted on her responses then, and now as an adult. The formulation diagram (Fig. 6.3) shows Tatenda's thoughts and feelings rated with an intensity level. In terms of prioritising care, the thoughts that have a higher intensity and are more 'hot-wired' to her current state of emotional distress would be prioritised for assessment and interventions (we look at this under the 'Plan' section). As part of the formulation, there is a need to consider which other theories may explain Tatenda's experience of distress. This will enable a mental health nurse and Tatenda to collaboratively consider Tatenda's experiences more holistically.

WHICH UNDERPINNING THEORIES TO EXPLORE AS PART OF TATENDA'S FORMULATION

There are a number of theories that could be drawn upon to understand Tatenda's experience of distress and her use of substances. Let us explore a few of these and how a mental health nurse might collaborate with Tatenda to help make sense of the distress she is experiencing.

Attachment Theory

Drawing on Tatenda's early life experiences, her father was not home much due to his work with the army. What has become known as 'conventional' attachment theory, (that is dominant attachment theory understanding) would ascribe a particular outcome or pathway as an emergent character of individuals for whom these 'absences' were central to their formative years. Bowlby's Attachment Theory for example, which is addressed in other chapters of this book, is viewed as seminal in this regard. However, culture plays a significant role in the variations observed in the manifestation, expression and meaning of attachment behaviours. One of the criticisms of attachment theory is that it is too reductionist and fails to consider the complexities of human subjectivity (Fonagy & Campbell, 2015) or family complexities and variations such as culture and environment. For instance, in Africa, where multiple cultures coexist,

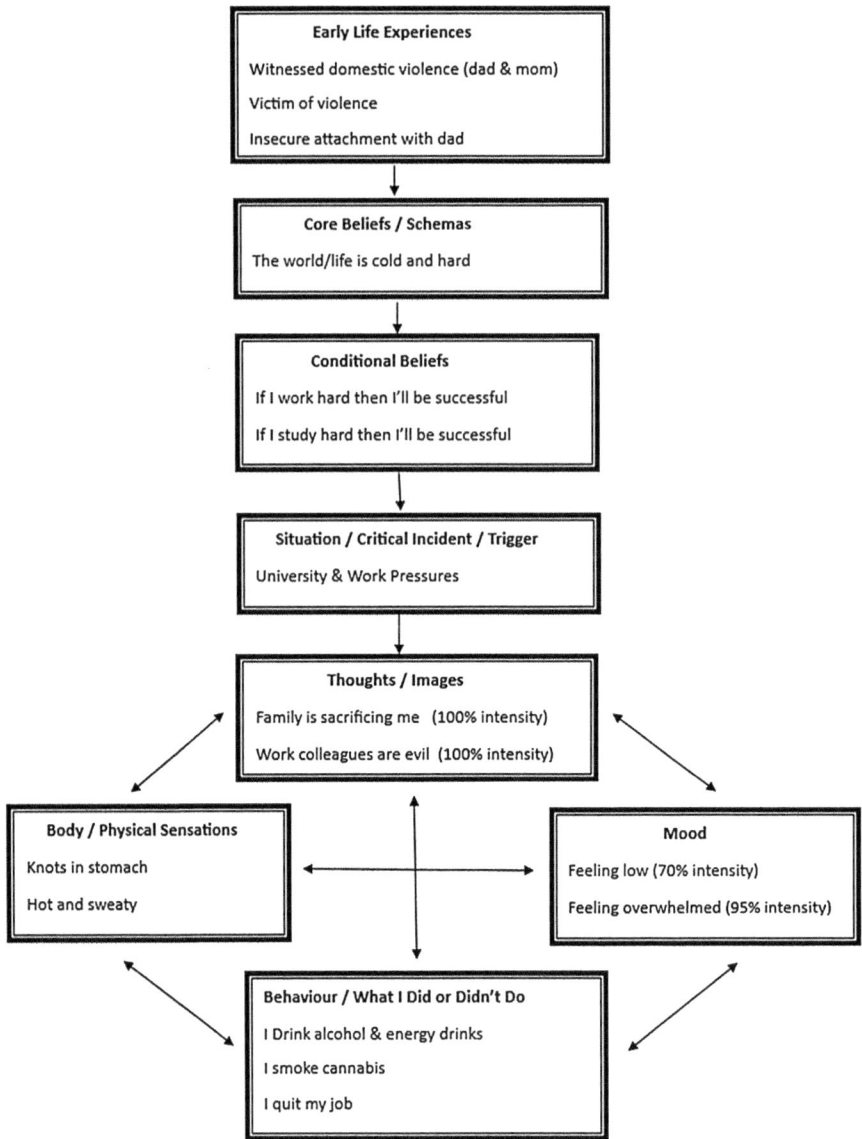

Fig. 6.3 Tatenda's Longitudinal CBT Formulation

there are distinct organisations of caregiving relationships underlying the development of attachment (Voges et al., 2019). The central and much more active role of the extended family for instance, means that there can be, and are, numerous parental figures to whom a child can be securely attached (even if attachment with a father, as in Tatenda's example, may have been 'insecure'). The parental role is often distributed across several individuals who may even be referred to using the same relational title, for example, the mother's sisters in Zimbabwean culture are often referred to as mum/mother rather than aunt. This affordance of the mother title is not just referential but is imbued with the same (sometimes higher) levels of connection. Aunts (also referred to as mothers) are often viewed as more approachable and therefore it is not uncommon for children to form stronger bonds with their aunts as opposed to their biological mothers. This, even in healthy family units that are not characterised by any form of trauma, may lead children to become attached to other people who are not their biological family. This extends also to uncles (father's brothers or mother's brothers) who also can be and are parental figures. Contrary to this being viewed as 'diluting' attachment, these extensions often enhance a sense of security for the children as they develop. Traditional and customary lines of responsibility, which are a form of African will practices—often elect a particular person as the default parental figure in the event of death of biological parents. Typically, this individual becomes an actively present person in the children's lives getting to know them and connect with them, akin to the 'God parent' role in western societies. Attachments form between these individuals and children and they become a central figure in the children's formative years. In Tatenda's case, it is therefore essential to position her relationship with her aunt as a very strong protective factor against the effects that dominant attachment theory identifies in response to the father's absences. One of the useful approaches would be to work with Tatenda to put together a family tree that may help to bring into sharp focus, the family structures that she can tap into for support. Anchoring herself to the extended family structure could play a significant role in her sense of worth and belonging, given her (dis)location currently.

Theory on Dual Diagnosis

Tatenda is experiencing co-occurring substance use and a struggle with her mental health. The literature refers to this as dual diagnosis, which is an ambiguous term, as essentially having any two diagnoses could also be viewed as dual diagnosis. However, for purposes of establishing and recognising that some individuals may have experiences of co-occurring mental health and substance use, dual diagnosis offers some theories that explain the relationship between the mental health and the substance use. While substance or alcohol use and emotional distress may initially be unrelated, over time they can interact and become mutually sustaining. Some theories on dual diagnosis include

- Self-Medicating Theory: Primary mental health problems may instigate the use of substances, for example as a coping strategy or method of self-medicating
- Causality Theory: Substance use and/or withdrawal leads to psychiatric symptoms or illness. Or a psychiatric problem can be caused or exacerbated by substance use, for example substance induced psychosis

- Multiple Risk Factor Theory: Multiple factors that may contribute to the experience of emotional distress and substance use, for example living in areas of high drug/alcohol use and having access to drugs/alcohol, social isolation, poverty, lack of responsible adult role models, suffering from traumatic life events.
- Super Sensitivity Theory: Combination of risk factors including psycho-biological vulnerability, interaction with environmental stress which can precipitate relapse or onset of emotional distress.
- Substance misuse and mental health problem that do not appear related (DH, 2009)

Assessing whether Tatenda's cannabis and alcohol use are related or interacting with her emotional distress would be helpful for informing intervention planning. For example, if her emotional distress (psychosis) is substance induced, then the approach to support and treatment would include Tatenda having a programme of care to help her stop using cannabis and alcohol, which may see an improvement in her emotional distress. If however, there are other underlying factors that have contributed to her use of substances, then the plan of care would need to be adjusted accordingly. The relationship is not an easy one to establish, but a useful starting point would be a comprehensive and collaborative assessment that then draws on theories to support the formulation. Tatenda may be reluctant to discuss her cannabis and alcohol use. As part of formulation, recognition of the wider context can help to understand her thoughts and feelings around this; as we know, substance use may have legal ramifications (e.g. cannabis is currently a Class B drug in the UK). Bearing in mind that if Tatenda was living in a different country (e.g. at the time of writing this chapter, in Canada, cannabis legality is different to the UK), there would be a need for a mental health nurse to provide support in line with that environment and its laws. A collaborative formulation that also involves the multidisciplinary team (MDT) is also helpful, particularly because different positionalities allow for a wide range of perspectives to be used to inform holistic interventions. The psychiatrist might respond to feelings of depression of individuals who struggle with alcohol use with medication or therapy, without exploring the connections between the person's drinking and their feelings (maybe forgetting that alcohol itself is a depressant that suppresses the central nervous system). A social worker might see environmental factors such as unemployment, poverty, racism, homophobia which may be part of an individual's life experience. The family therapist might identify patterns of communication that feed the cycle of shame and blame that family members might perpetuate. Meanwhile, the pastoral counsellor may see a spiritual crisis that has compromised the individual's values, belief system and self-worth. Collectively, professionals can support with consideration of multifaceted contributory factors and presentations.

Trauma Theory

The Indicative Trauma Impact Manual (ITIM) by Taylor and Shrive (2023) outlines the importance of reflecting on, exploring, examining and understanding the role that trauma can play in mental health and where individuals use substances. Taylor and Shrive (2023) outline various distressing or traumatic experiences and then explore trauma responses, which are often about self-preservation, and adaptations to stimuli from the lens of learnt behaviour. The key considerations here are that self-preservation is 'normal', and adaptation is 'normal'—as human beings, these adaptations are vital for our survival. Giving the example of self-preservation, we follow a course of action in life to ensure our survival, and if introduced to environments or conditions we are unfamiliar with, whether these are nurturing or challenging, we adapt to the circumstances. Tatenda witnessed her father's violence against her mother, and she was a victim of her father's violence. Tatenda has also experienced domestic violence in her marital home. It is common for people who experience violence or assaults to have longlasting trauma responses and it is therefore important to remain non-judgemental (Taylor & Shrive, 2023).

Tatenda went to boarding school and this too is recognised in the ITIM as a source of trauma which can trigger a sense of loss, separation or disconnection from family, and the highly structured environment can contribute to feelings of powerlessness for some. Other potential traumas that Tatenda has experienced include post-migration challenges associated with her relocation from Gokwe, Zimbabwe to London, UK, being far from friends and extended family and finding the only option available to her to make ends meet was to work as a prostitute. Additionally, the loss of her mother and sibling at age 11 are areas that the mental health nurse would sensitively explore through formulation to understand the links that these may have with her current emotional distress and use of substances. The difficulty we may have in nursing is that we are accustomed to referring to use of alcohol or self-harm to cope as 'maladaptive coping strategies'. This concept can be particularly challenging as it labels the coping strategy as 'negative' without considering the trauma context in which the coping strategy developed. While the goal may be to support Tatenda to explore alternative ways of managing her emotional distress, the mental health nurse undertaking formulation would need to be mindful of the language they use, and recognise that Tatenda's current coping strategies can be positioned as understandable given her personal circumstances.

Theory on Loss

Tatenda has experienced a significant number of losses during her childhood as well as in adulthood. Theory on loss can help the exploration of this. Bowlby (1980) developed a theory of loss, grief, and mourning that remains the most referred to, the theory brings together attachment theory and case studies. The clinical application of theories demands a very intentional, deliberate recognition of the context from which individuals come to experience and process loss. There is need to heed the nuances and peculiarities of each situation and respond with an acknowledgement of its uniqueness. Particularly, how different societies perceive loss and the sense-making processes they employ in their navigation of loss. Central to this, is the role and function of surrounding conditions, community values and belief systems. Different societies and communities experience the impact of a death in the family in different ways that are socially constructed by their cultural experiences and perspectives. Such experiences and perspectives cannot be universalised (Radzilani, 2010).

As Tatenda is African, it is important to consider some African theoretical frameworks in relation to loss. One such framework is Nwoye's African Grief perspective on grieving and mourning. This perspective identifies the process of grieving as active work rather than a passive process that happens to someone who in turn suffers its effects. African grief work is defined as the patterns inscribed in traditional communities for successful healing of the psychological wounds and the easing of the painful burden of loss (Nwoye, 2005; Sisodia, 1997). This perspective focuses on the spiritual, systematic and interactional nature of healing in grieving and the resources that the community makes available to bereaved individuals (Nwoye, 2005). African grief perspective is rooted in three interrelated objectives; firstly, to engage in activities that mitigate the impact of loss; secondly, to safeguard the bereaved from extreme suffering as a result of their loss; and finally, to avail bereavement rituals approved by the community, designed to help the bereaved put grief into context with an understanding and acceptance that there is hope after grief (Makgahlela, 2016; Nwoye, 2005). These grieving rituals extend beyond grieving in relation to death; for example loss of relationships also carries particular practices designed to bring a sense of closure to both parties.

In most African communities, tradition plays a significant role in the day-to-day routines of individuals—as a vital aspect of identity, values, and norms. Within this context, the reaction to death is influenced by how death is assimilated into a specific culture (Appel, 2011). Generally, Africans believe that death completes an elaborate life cycle, is accepted as a rite of passage to the spiritual realm, away from the physicality of this life (Cebekhulu, 2016; Rugonye & Bukaliya, 2016). Thus, reaching out to, and communication with deceased people is understood as a natural connection and not pathologised in the ways that western understandings of communication with deceased are often viewed. Making room for the possibility of communication with a deceased person forms part of the healing process, with relief drawn from the belief of continued 'accessibility' despite physical separation through death. This is not to say that tradition and culture is not sometimes problematic, rather a call for balance and objectivity as opposed to uncritically defaulting to narrow understandings.

Culturally Responsive Trauma Informed Care (TIC)

One aspect of formulation is, of course, ethnicity and culture. Johnstone and Dallos (2014) ask a series of questions such as: how can we ensure that cultural identities and values are fully incorporated into the process of formulation? And what constitutes a 'problem' as opposed to a cultural variation in acceptable behaviour? More generally, formulation is itself a concept that has arisen within a particular culture. To what extent does this limit its usefulness beyond that culture, and is there any way of compensating for this? TIC is defined as organisational or care system's culture and policy-backed structure; interventions and direct practice approaches (Bateman & Henderson, 2013) that encompass several common elements or principles. Substance Abuse and Mental Health Services Administration (SAMHSA) (2014) argues that six key principles should be in place to ensure a care is sensitive and responsive to the traumas that patients have experienced in their lives. Namely: safety; trustworthiness and transparency; peer support; collaboration and mutuality; empowerment, voice, and choice; and cultural, historical, and gender issues. TIC must be inclusive, centring patient and family collaboration with practitioners (Elliott et al., 2005).

Given the information in the case study, some of the trauma that Tatenda could be living with may relate to varying conceptualisations of effective and acceptable discipline and what was normalised in marital relationships. Non-western or culturally unique ways of coping and responding to trauma are often unrecognised or unattended to in mainstream systems, so culturally responsive and relevant assessment or service options for migrant populations are often non-existent (Asgary & Segar 2011; Colucci et al., 2015; Morris et al., 2009). Although unlikely to be explicitly included in every health formulation, the process should include an attempt to understand the health beliefs and explanatory systems of the individual in the context of the historically, socially and culturally specific constructs of illness and health that the individual lives within—including any apparent health norms related to ascribed characteristics such as gender, race, ethnicity, and class—and how these sit with wider discourses about health and illness within any minority or socially marginalised groups that the individual might personally identify with, or be identified with by others (Cole, 2014).

Role of Religion

Within the Zimbabwean context, churches often function as psycho-social support through providing social connections and actively shaping individual behaviour and what is deemed acceptable presentation (Muswerakuenda et al., 2023). In terms of emotional health, research has shown that the church, prayer and the word of the bible can offer some congregants a sense of belonging, positive wellbeing and community (Burrell, 2021). Woodruff and Frakt (2020) purport however that the church and other religious-affiliated organisations have promising yet underexplored potential to provide social support services for treating substance use in communities where substance use treatment services are limited. This is noteworthy given the tendencies particularly with western societies to pathologise cultures and religions and what that means for helping individuals whose source of support and wellbeing may be religion and 'home' culture. For example, appropriation of blame for behaviour and presentation onto a 'demon' allows for the individual navigating substance use disorder—to be viewed more sympathetically as one tormented by an evil spirit, rather than being personally vilified. This has implications for the issue of stigma and how this manifests in the context of the individual's self-esteem. This perspective positions the individual as one who requires help and support to rid themselves of the 'demon' as opposed to an individual making poor personal choices. Supporting the person to be well and free from evil spirits thus becomes a communal goal shared and taken up by the church community. 'Collectivist' or community-based approaches to problem solving are embedded in many African cultures and captured through common proverbs such as, '*it takes a village to raise a child*' which emphasises the role of community support in shaping and moulding, disease prevention and management.

By contrast western health models are often 'individualistic' and person centred in a way that can further isolate individuals who are more accustomed to collectivist norms. More recently, however, the adaptation of principles such as social prescribing has begun to recognise the importance and need to work with the communities within which people reside, as more effective and sustainable sources of support. NHS England and Royal College of General Practitioners (2017) defined social prescribing as a way of linking patients in primary care with sources of support within the community. Social prescribing provides General Practitioners (GPs) with a non-medical referral option that can operate alongside existing treatments to improve health and wellbeing and are being widely promoted and adopted. Schemes commonly use services provided by the voluntary and community sector and can include an extensive range of practical information and advice, community activity, physical activities befriending and enabling services. Such services under the rubric of social prescribing are being described as a radical rethink to the provision of health and wellbeing services, making better use of community support structures and financially more sustainable.

Reduced number of health professionals has meant that Zimbabwe long recognised the importance of community-based interventions well before it was named social prescribing. Dixon Chibanda's Friendship Bench concept in Zimbabwe being a case in point. Chibanda a psychiatrist in Zimbabwe coined this intervention which is now recognised globally as an effective community-based intervention to support people who are struggling with their mental health. The Friendship Bench project in Zimbabwe engages the wider community through structured processes in wellbeing support for psychiatric patients (Centre for Global Mental Health, 2016). The community support comes in the form of elderly Zimbabwean women whose age and gender as cultural identity markers present them as safe, wise and trustworthy (Chibanda, 2006). These elderly women are affectionately known as the community grandmothers. These community grandmothers are, in the main, lay people who will have engaged in basic training with the hospitals to ensure cohesive support (Chibanda et al., 2017). The community support centres on providing the patient with hope and an opportunity to recalibrate their lives. This extension of patient support to the community further focuses the nurses' role on what are considered more clinical interventions. This is also a prime example of decolonising therapy and diversifying who as a global society we choose to learn from and whose knowledge we value. In Tatenda's case, as a person born and raised in Zimbabwe, interventions such as this may be more culturally appropriate, effective and sustainable.

It would be remiss to not highlight that conversely, communities can exacerbate individual challenges. For example, the church's expectation of what is acceptable behaviour within what are viewed as sacred spaces—can by contrast marginalise and further stigmatise individuals affected by substance use disorder. Hence the role and function of the church can be conflicted and contradictory, embracing and casting out at different junctures. Families too can support or reject at different points and sometimes simultaneously. The issue of 'shame' being central to the continuum along which support and acceptance is offered at various points.

Tatenda has thoughts about her family sacrificing her and that colleagues are evil. On the surface these may be experiences that others around her cannot relate to, however when working in a trauma informed way, there is need to consider that delusions can be a response to trauma for some individuals. Trauma can affect perception of reality and the delusions themselves are a coping strategy for the overwhelming emotions associated with trauma. Exploring and validating these experiences is key (Taylor & Shrive, 2023). It is worth exploring the link with the theme of religion with the notion of 'evil' and 'sacrifice' as these are aspects that would be found in the bible as an example. Exploring religion and church in a structured way and allowing it to be integrated as a possible protective factor when engaged with productively is worth considering as a framework through which hope can be nurtured for Tatenda.

PLAN

The planning stage of the nursing process provides an opportunity to set goals and recommend interventions which will support Tatenda with regard to her substance use and emotional distress. As a stage, it relies on information gathered at assessment, and the formulation developed. Planning (which involves goal setting) is a fundamental nursing skill, and Barrett et al. (2019) outline that a plan of care should have goals that are patient centred, recordable, observable/measurable, directive, understandable/clear, credible and time-related (PRODUCT). If a baseline establishes that Tatenda has specific areas of need regarding her health, then a goal would be aimed at helping Tatenda progress towards where she would like to be with her health and wellbeing. Farrelly et al. (2016) note that care plans are often not individualised to the specific patient and are mostly completed to meet organisational requirements. The mental health nurse can co-develop with Tatenda, a plan of care based on the information gathered at assessment, and the theoretically underpinned formulation. The plan of care would also consider the theories explored in the formulation, and the wider literature around these. For Tatenda, this would mean thinking about what interventions would be trauma informed, culturally sensitive and respectful of aspects to do with religion. Burrell (2021) notes that different cultures may understand and speak about mental health differently and it is important to recognise these differences, particularly when it comes to treatment options.

The appropriateness of a CBT Longitudinal Formulation as a basis to generate recommendations for treatment approaches should be critically analysed. Most therapies we know and use today are Eurocentric and were researched/conceived in the nineteenth and twentieth centuries where issues of racism, colonialism, oppression and disenfranchisement of certain people were rife, and there needs to be consideration of whether these therapies in their original form are helpful for a diverse range of individuals (Zahid, 2021). Burrell (2021) notes that therapy or treatment options that are based on European views of the nature of humanity may lack relevance to non-Europeans. Bignall et al., (2019) suggest the need to provide treatment therapies that are more culturally sensitive to enable inclusive approaches to treatment.

With the above in mind, pharmacotherapy might be recommended together with CBT to help with Tatenda's thoughts, feelings of being overwhelmed constantly and her substance use (see formulation Fig. 6.3). In the UK, this would be aligned to NICE Clinical guideline [CG178] which recommends the use of psychotherapies such as CBT in conjunction with antipsychotic medication for first episode psychosis (NICE, 2014). However, considerations could be given to a culturally adapted version of CBT (Rathod et al., 2013). This is because if used in its original form, its individualistic values and emphasis on rational thinking can be interpreted in ways that might devalue Tatenda's culture that esteems collectivism and spirituality respectively. This may not fully meet Tatenda's needs and may inadvertently result in her disengaging from treatment or services, especially if Tatenda has a sense that CBT and the mental health nurse or therapist does not embrace, appreciate her diversity, understand where she is coming from, or her sense of identity. It is promising to see that within the last few years, there has been a concerted effort to undertake research on adapting existing therapies to develop an evidence base for their effectiveness. For example there is a growing evidence base on culturally adapted CBT and culturally adapted therapeutic approaches such as counselling, and these will contribute to enhancing mental health or substance use support for individuals from cultures that value collectivism. The research has largely focussed on adjusting awareness of relevant cultural factors and therapy preparation;

assessment and engagement; and adjustments in therapy (Naeem et al., 2015). While a mental health nurse may not deliver CBT (unless trained), an awareness of, and ability to engage appropriately with individuals from diverse cultures would not only demonstrate valuing of difference but would enhance the therapeutic nurse-patient relationship as an important step for building trust with Tatenda.

IMPLEMENT

Implementing planned care is another key part of the nursing process. This stage involves carrying out the interventions that are outlined in the plan of care. Barrett et al. (2019) identify some helpful questions to guide implementation, such as whether the care is person centred, safe, legal and ethical, whether it is evidence-based, and whether there are the required resources to provide the recommended care. Other important questions to consider include patient consent, quality of communication and documentation of the delivery of the interventions. During the implementation stage, some challenges may arise if the planned care (in this case culturally adapted CBT for Tatenda) is not implemented as planned. Due to the multiple losses Tatenda has experienced some of the trauma associated may resurface so it is important to approach interventions with sensitivity and compassion. Consideration can be made around any anniversaries when Tatenda experienced loss, like the passing of her mother. The periods before the anniversary and after the anniversary are also potentially vulnerable moments for Tatenda, so these should be considered when implementing interventions and reviewing her engagement.

Mental health nurses in spaces where they interact with individuals experiencing distress are well positioned to provide therapeutic support. While not all mental health nurses will have training on specific therapies such as CBT or counselling, they are skilled in building therapeutic helping relationships. The conversations and interactions that happen outside of the intervention implementation are also very important, and the formulation developed can inform what support looks like. Nkansa-Dwamena (2017) highlights that learning, practising, and communicating in a way that understands and empathises with factors related to diversity and inclusion is important, and this is true for any helping profession. For the mental health nursing professional who spends comparably more time with individuals in distress (e.g. 24-hr care on ward settings), this opens up possibilities for enhancing the therapeutic role, and ultimately the potential for helping individuals in distress during the intervention implementation stage.

EVALUATE

Evaluate is the final stage of the nursing process which involves reviewing whether the interventions have helped an individual as planned, and whether the interventions were realistic and achievable (considering any factors that may come to light during implementation). This stage allows for the nurse and patient to review whether the resources to facilitate the interventions were sufficient, and if there is a need to continue with the current interventions, or if new goals need to be set (triggering the cycle of assessment planning implementation and evaluation again). If the desired goals set in the care plan are achieved (in Tatenda's example, a reduction/stopping alcohol and cannabis consumption, and relief from the symptoms of her emotional distress), then the plan of care and interventions will have been successful at meeting her needs. Sometimes evaluation may reveal partial success or no success at all—this does not represent a failure, but just a need to re-evaluate goals, resources and explore if there were any unidentified factors that might have hindered recovery so that a plan can be made to incorporate these into any revised approaches for support.

In summary, based on Tatenda's formulation it is important to consider her holistically, which includes her culture and ethnicity as these may have a bearing on her worldview, and may enable a better understanding of her experiences of distress so as to adapt and tailor interventions around her needs. Formulation by its very nature prompts these considerations. The UK offers a rich and multi-cultural environment; however, recent reviews of literature indicate that services or interventions are not designed with cultural diversity in mind, and this can be a barrier to individuals accessing mental health support and treatment (Nwokoroku et al., 2022). This review also acknowledges that '*One therapeutic model cannot serve all in a culturally diverse society such as the UK*', and as such it invites the opportunity for working with ethnic minority communities in designing services that are more inclusive. There are training implications—to be able to practise in a more culturally sensitive and culturally competent way. Professionals need to be able to engage with cultural diversity in a more meaningful way, and to value different ways of knowing or thinking to be able to support those in distress from different cultural backgrounds. We hope that this chapter has stimulated thinking around how formulation can and should consider the whole person, especially where their culture and spirituality are significant parts of their experience and identity. We have explored the role that the mental health nurse can play through embedding principles of formulation within day-to-day practice and the nursing process. While we have explored some potential theories and considerations that would be central to Tatenda's formulation, it is important to acknowledge that there are a range of other theories that could be equally useful to draw upon. The main consideration for a nurse is that they are drawing on theory that can help make sense of the individual's experience of distress, and then collaboratively (with the patient) plan and deliver interventions that are tailored to the individual's needs and supports their journey towards recovery.

Points for Reflection
1. Reflect on some of the dominant theories you are aware of in any area of mental health (e.g. theories on psychosis). Then delve into the literature to explore what other theories exist—consider theories that spotlight various cultural perspectives and different explanatory systems.
2. Consider what your own positioning is with regard to religion and spirituality—have you come across situations where religion was an important part of supporting an individual you were working with and if so, in what ways did you provide support?
3. Reflect on what your takeaway is from this chapter and make note of at least one thing that you would like to do differently (or to continue doing) in practice following reading this chapter.

References

Appel, D. L. (2011). Narratives on death and bereavement from three South African Cultures. *Journal of Psychology in Africa, 23*(3), 453–458. https://doi.org/10.1080/14330237.2013.10820651

Asgary, R., & Segar, N. (2011). Barriers to health care access among refugee asylum seekers. *Journal of Health Care for the Poor and Underserved, 22,* 506–522.

Assadi, G. (2020). The mental state examination. *British Journal of Nursing.* Mark Allen Group, *29*(22), 1328–1332. https://doi.org/10.12968/bjon.2020.29.22.1328

Bakke, O. (2018). WHO Launches Global status report on alcohol and health 2018. Available: www.add-resources.org. World Health Organization.

Barrett, D., Wilson, B., & Woollands, A. (2019). *Care planning: A guide for nurses* (3rd ed.). Routledge. https://doi.org/10.4324/9781315630106

Bateman, J., & Henderson, C. (2013). *Trauma-informed care and practice: Towards a cultural shift in policy reform across mental health and human services in Australia – A national strategic direction.* Mental Health Coordinating Council: Rozelle.

Bignall, T., Jeraj, S., Helsby, E., & Butt, J. (2019). *Racial disparities in mental health.* London: Race Equity Foundation.

Borrell-Carrió, F., Suchman, A. L., & Epstein, R. M. (2004). The biopsychosocial model 25 years later: Principles, practice, and scientific inquiry. *Annals of Family Medicine., 2*(6), 576–582. https://doi.org/10.1370/afm.245

Bowlby, J. (1980). *Attachment and Loss, Vol. 3: Loss: Sadness and Depression.* London: Hogarth Press and Institute of Psycho-Analysis.

British Psychological Society. (2011). Good practice guidelines on the use of psychological formulation. *The British Psychological Society.* https://doi.org/10.53841/bpsrep.2011.rep100

Buescher, T., & McGugan, S. (2022). Standing out on the margins: Using dialogical narrative analysis to explore mental health student nurse identity construction and core modules. *Issues in Mental Health Nursing, 43*(8), 737–747. https://doi.org/10.1080/01612840.2022.2037174

Burrell, R. R. (2021). Religion, therapy and mental health treatment in diverse communities: Some critical reflections and radical propositions, chapter 18 p. 199–212. In Charura, D and Lago, C (eds.). *Black Identities and White Therapies: Race, Respect and Diversity*. PCCS Books Ltd.

Cebekhulu, L. M. (2016). Understanding the experiences of young widows in rural KwaZuluNatal: University of Kwazulu-Natal. [Masters dissertation].

Centre for Global Mental Health. (2016). The Friendship Bench. [Online]. Retrieved October 4, 2020, from https://www.centreforglobalmentalhealth.org/the-friendship-bench

Chibanda, D. (2006). The Friendship Bench. [Online]. Retrieved October 4, 2023, from https://www.friendshipbenchzimbabwe.org/

Chibanda, D., Cowan, F., Verhey, R., Machando, D., Abas, M., & Lund, C. (2017). Lay health workers' experience of delivering a problem solving therapy intervention for common mental disorders among people living with HIV: A qualitative study from Zimbabwe. *Community Mental Health Journal., 53*(2), 143–153.

Coffey, M., Cohen, R., Faulkner, A., Hannigan, B., Simpson, A., & Barlow, S. (2017). Ordinary risks and accepted fictions: How contrasting and competing priorities work in risk assessment and mental health care planning. *Health Expectations, 20*(3), 471–483. https://doi.org/10.1111/hex.12474

Cole. (2014). Using integrative formulation in health setting. In Johnstone, L. & Dallos, R. (eds.) *Formulation in Psychology and Psychotherapy Making Sense of People's Problems*. London: Routledge.

Colucci, E., Minas, H., Szwarc, J., Guerra, C., & Paxton, G. (2015). In or out? Barriers and facilitators to refugee-background young people accessing mental health services. *Transcult. Psychiatry, 52*, 766–790.

Department of Health. (2009). *Signs for improvement: Commissioning interventions to reduce alcohol related harm*. London: Department of Health.

Department of Health. (2016). Alcohol guidelines review – Report from the guidelines development group to the UK Chief Medical Officers. Department of Health. Available: https://assets.publishing.service.gov.uk/government/uploads/system/uploads/attachment_data/file/545739/GDG_report-Jan2016.pdf

Earnshaw, V. (2020). Stigma and substance use disorders: A clinical, research, and advocacy agenda. *Am Psychol., 75*(9), 1300–1311. https://doi.org/10.1037/amp0000744

Elliott, D., Bjelajac, P., Fallot, R. D., Markoff, L. S., & Reed, B. G. (2005). Trauma-informed or Trauma-denied: Principles and Implementation of Trauma-informed Services for Women. *Wiley Online Library, 33*, 461–477.

Engel, G. L. (1977). The need for a new medical model: A challenge for biomedicine. *Science, 196*(4286), 129–136.

Farrelly, S., Lester, H., Rose, D., Birchwood, M., Marshall, M., Waheed, W., Henderson, R. C., Szmukler, G., & Thornicroft, G. (2016). Barriers to shared decision making in mental health care: Qualitative study of the Joint Crisis Plan for psychosis. *Health Expectations: An International Journal of Public Participation in Health Care and Health Policy, 19*(2), 448–458. https://doi.org/10.1111/hex.12368

Fonagy, P., & Campbell, C. (2015). Bad blood revisited: Attachment and psychoanalysis, 2015. *British Journal of Psychotherapy, 31*(2), 229–250. https://doi.org/10.1111/bjp.12150

Foster, K., Marks, P., O'Brien, A., & Raeburn, T. (2020). *Mental health in nursing: Theory and practice for clinical settings* (5th ed.). Elsevier Health Sciences.

Goldberg, D., & Murray, R. (2002). *The maudsley handbook of practical psychiatry* (4th edition). Oxford University Press.

Hall, W. (1997). The role of legal coercion in the treatment of offenders with alcohol and heroin problems. *Australian and New Zealand Journal of Criminology, 30*, 103–120. https://doi.org/10.1177/0004865897030002

Harkins, C., Morleo, M., Cook, P. A., & Bellis, M. A. (2010). *Understanding the views of healthcare professionals towards alcohol consumption and the provision of alcohol advice*. Drinkwise Northwest Centre for Public Health & Liverpool John Moores University.

Institute of Alcohol Studies. (2023). Language bank: Talking about inequalities in alcohol use and harm. Retrieved March 10, 2024, from https://www.ias.org.uk/wp-content/uploads/2023/11/Language-Bank-Talking-About-Inequalities-in-Alcohol-Use-and-Harm.pdf

Johnstone, L., & Dallos, R. (2006). *Formulation in psychology and psychotherapy: Making sense of people's problems*. Routledge. https://doi.org/10.4324/9780203087268

Johnstone, L., & Dallos, R. (2014). Introduction to formulation (chapter 1). In Johnstone, L. & Dallos, R. (eds) *Formulation in Psychology and Psychotherapy Making Sense of People's Problems*. London: Routledge.

Kaya, G. K., Ward, J. R., & Clarkson, P. J. (2019). A framework to support risk assessment in hospitals. *International Journal for Quality in Health Care, 31*(5), 393–401. https://doi.org/10.1093/intqhc/mzy194

Makgahlela, M. W. (2016). The psychology of bereavement and mourning rituals in a Northern Sotho community. Doctoral dissertation, University of Limpopo.

McClelland, L. (2014). Reformulating the impact of social inequalities. Power and Social Justice (Chapter 6). In Johnstone, L. & Dallos, R. (eds) *Formulation in Psychology and Psychotherapy Making Sense of People's Problems*. London: Routledge.

Morris, M., Popper, S., Rodwell, T., Brodine, S., & Brouwer, K. (2009). Healthcare barriers of refugees post-resettlement. *Journal of Community Health, 34*, 529–538.

Muswerakuenda, F. F., Mundagowa, P. T., Madziwa, C., & Mukora-Mutseyekwa, F. (2023). Access to psychosocial support for church-going young people recovering from drug and substance abuse in zimbabwe: A qualitative study. *BMC Public Health, 23*(1), 723. https://doi.org/10.1186/s12889-023-15633-8

Naeem, F., Phiri, P., Munshi, T., Rathod, S., Ayub, M., Gobbi, M., & Kingdon, D. (2015). Using cognitive behaviour therapy with South Asian Muslims: Findings from the culturally sensitive CBT project. *International Review of Psychiatry, 27*(3), 233–246. https://doi.org/10.3109/09540261.2015.1067598

National Institute for Health and Care Excellence. (2011). *Coexisting severe mental illness (psychosis) and substance misuse: assessment and management in healthcare settings | Guidance [CG120]*. NICE. Retrieved December 29, 2020, from https://www.nice.org.uk/guidance/CG120/chapter/1-Guidance#recognition-of-psychosis-with-coexisting-substance-misuse

National Institute for Health and Care Excellence. (2014). *Psychosis and schizophrenia in adults: Prevention and management. [CG178]*. NICE. https://www.nice.org.uk/guidance/cg178/resources/psychosis-and-schizophrenia-in-adults-prevention-and-management-pdf-35109758952133

NHS England and Royal College of General Practitioners. (2017). General Practice Forward Review. [Online]. Retrieved October 4, 2023, from https://www.england.nhs.uk/wp-content/uploads/2016/04/gpfv.pdf

Nkansa-Dwamena, O. (2017). Issues of race and ethnicity in counselling psychology, Chapter 18. In J. Murphy (Ed.), *Counselling psychology: A textbook for study and practice*. John Wiley & Sons Ltd.

Nursing and Midwifery Council. (2018). Future nurse: Standards of proficiency for registered nurses. https://www.nmc.org.uk/globalassets/sitedocuments/education-standards/future-nurse-proficiencies.pdf

Nwokoroku, S. C., Neil, B., Dlamini, C., & Osuchukwu, V. C. (2022). A systematic review of the role of culture in the mental health service utilisation among ethnic minority groups in the United Kingdom. *Global Mental Health*, *9*, 84–93. https://doi.org/10.1017/gmh.2022.2

Nwoye, A. (2005). Memory healing processes and community intervention in grief work in Africa. *Australian and New Zealand Journal of Family Therapy*, *26*(3), 147–154. https://doi.org/10.1002/j.1467-8438.2005.tb00662.x

Obot, I. S., & Room, R. (2005). *Alcohol gender and drinking problems: Perspectives from low and middle-income countries*. Geneva: World Health Organization. http://www.who.int/substance_abuse/publications/alcohol_gender_drinking_problems.pdf

Pycroft, A. (2010). *Understanding & working with substance misusers*. SAGE. https://doi.org/10.4135/9781446251331

Radzilani, M. S. (2010). A discourse analysis of bereavement rituals in a Tshivenda speaking community: African Christian and Traditional African perceptions. Doctoral dissertation, University of Pretoria.

Rathod, S., Phiri, P., Harris, S., Underwood, C., Thagadur, M., Padmanabi, U., & Kingdon, D. (2013). Cognitive behaviour therapy for psychosis can be adapted for minority ethnic groups: A randomised controlled trial. *Schizophrenia Research*, *143*(2), 319–326. https://doi.org/10.1016/j.schres.2012.11.007

Rugonye, S., & Bukaliya, R. (2016). Effectiveness of the African bereavement counselling techniques: A case of Shona people of Zimbabwe: Implications for open and distance learning institutions. *International Journal of Humanities Social Sciences and Education*, *3*(2), 49–56.

Sisodia, I. D. (1997). New horizons in systemic family therapy. November meeting of the World Council for Psychotherapy Held in Kampala, 23, 1.

Substance Abuse and Mental Health Services Administration. (2014). *SAMHSA's concept of trauma and guidance for a trauma-informed approach*. SAMSHA.

Taylor, J., & Shrive, J. (2023). *Indicative Trauma Impact Manual: A non-diagnostic, trauma informed guide to emotion, thought, and behaviour* (1st ed.). VictimFocus.

Voges, J., Berg, A., & Niehaus, D. J. H. (2019). Revisiting the African origins of attachment research - 50 years on from Ainsworth: A descriptive review. *Infant Mental Health Journal*, *40*(6): 799–816. https://doi.org/10.1002/imhj.21821. Epub 2019 Aug 11. PMID: 31402473.

Warrender, D., Connell, C., Jones, E., Monteux, S., Colwell, L., Laker, C., & Cromar-Hayes, M. (2024). Mental health deserves better: Resisting the dilution of specialist pre-registration mental health nurse education in the united kingdom. *International Journal of Mental Health Nursing*, *33*(1), 202–212. https://doi.org/10.1111/inm.13236

Woodruff, A., & Frakt, A. B. (2020). Can churches bring addiction treatment to rural areas? *Health Affairs Forefront*. https://doi.org/10.1377/forefront.20200406.943992

World Health Organisation. (2022). *World mental health report: Transforming mental health for all*. World Health Organization.

World Health Organization. (2019). *The WHO special initiative for mental health (2019–2023): Universal health coverage for mental health*. World Health Organization. https://iris.who.int/handle/10665/310981

World Health Organization (WHO) and United Nations Office on Drugs and Crime (UNODC). (2020). *International standards for the treatment of drug use disorders: Revised edition incorporating results of field-testing*. WHO & UNODC.

Zahid, N. (2021). Lifting the white veil of therapy, chapter 10, p. 107–118. In Charura, D and Lago, C (eds.). *Black Identities and White Therapies: Race, Respect and Diversity*. PCCS Books Ltd.

CHAPTER 7

Formulation to Support Individuals Who Are Experiencing Emotional Distress and Associated Self-Harm

Lolita Alfred, Betty Williamson, and Charity Mudimu

Key Learning Points
- Seeing the whole person
- Emotional distress and self-harm through the lens of trauma
- Biopsychosocial collaborative formulation
- The importance of compassionate care and engendering hope
- The role of mental health nurses
- Opportunities for formulation within crisis and home treatment services

The following chapter begins with Betty's story—an anonymised account provided with Betty's consent. The chapter explores what a compassionate approach to listening, hearing and understanding the lived experience might look like, and it explores considerations for biopsychosocial formulation to support recovery. While Betty's experience was mainly with services such as accident and emergency, acute in-patient psychiatric hospital settings and general practice (GP) services, this chapter explores how formulation might be

L. Alfred (✉) • C. Mudimu
City, University of London, London, UK
e-mail: Lolita.Alfred@city.ac.uk; Charity.Mudimu@city.ac.uk

B. Williamson
London, UK

© The Author(s), under exclusive license to Springer Nature Switzerland AG 2024
V. Howard, L. Alfred (eds.), *Formulation in Mental Health Nursing*,
https://doi.org/10.1007/978-3-031-59956-9_7

approached in a different service such as the Home Treatment Team (HTT). It also considers the role of mental health nurses within the HTT, and as members of the multidisciplinary team.

Introducing Betty

I found self-harm as a way of managing overwhelming emotional distress quite by accident. It was the early 2000s and I was thrilled to be pregnant with a planned pregnancy. However, this joy quickly turned to despair as I found the pandora's box (which I had spent many years keeping the lid firmly fixed shut) was creeping open and becoming increasingly difficult to push back down. When we consider the biosocial model approach and the invalidation I had experienced. These memories and experiences were haunting me and my days were filled with vivid memories. As the pregnancy progressed in its early embryonic stages I questioned how I could provide a different experience for this child, and would I be able to keep him or her safe? I wrestled with my sub-conscious time and time again. I then slipped and had a fall whilst working as a hairdresser. Concerned about the impact on the pregnancy I was referred for an early scan where I was relieved to see a heartbeat. Sadly a few weeks later I started bleeding and all worries about 'could I keep the child safe', turned to 'just let the pregnancy survive'…But it didn't.

And so began my journey of self-harm a couple of months later. It began with me accidentally scratching myself whilst sewing. There was a moment of 'gosh that scratch provided an escape from the emotional distress'. Not only of my past, but the feelings of guilt in relation to losing the much-wanted pregnancy. The odd scratch or two quickly escalated to significant scratching until my arms were red raw and weeping. During this time the self-harm was akin to a release of a pressure cooker valve. My head was the pressure cooker, and it was overcome with emotional distress and pain. I found that as I cut, it felt like the blood that drained was intertwined with the emotional distress and the pain that came with it.

Within two months I was cutting using a Stanley knife from the toolbox and using the sharp knives from the kitchen. My descent into needing to cut firmer and deeper was rapid. During this time, I had my first admission into a psychiatric hospital. An old-style hospital which has long since been replaced by a new building. This curtailed the deep cutting briefly. However, during this admission I would search for anything remotely sharp to scratch myself with. During this admission, it became clear how traumatised I was. This resulted in my being referred to a clinical psychologist. This was incredibly painful as it was very much a talking therapy and going through deeply upsetting and distressing events in my life. My self-harm continued unabated. During the early 2000s I found there was limited understanding about how self-harm helped me, my Community Psychiatric Nurse was very much of the view that I should just stop it! However, no other strategies were offered to replace the self-harm. This resulted in conflict between myself and my Community Psychiatric Nurse which was incredibly painful for me. During this time, I was also overdosing with medication. This was a way of blocking out the memories which haunted me every day. I didn't want to die, but I didn't want the life I had either. I was referred to a day hospital to keep me safe at least during the daytime. Due to the overdoses a member of staff insisted that I bring my sleeping medication and other medication into the day centre each day and I was allowed the prescribed dose to take home with me each afternoon. I was also prescribed Prozac which made me significantly more poorly. The psychiatrist became frustrated with me after one of my overdoses. Their solution was to increase the Prozac, which sadly made me even more distressed. Once I was discharged from the day hospital, I gradually weaned myself off the Prozac as I was convinced it was making me more poorly. Mid 2000 I was relatively stable, and the self-harm was more under control.

Unfortunately, things came to a head, when I had an ectopic pregnancy and moved to a different area of the country. My descent back into self-harm was rapid. I was having to attend A&E on a regular basis and was fortunate to be referred to a Liaison Psychiatric nurse who was kind and specialised in self-harm. He saw the whole person, not just the self-harm and quickly set about identifying how best to support me. I still have the A4 workings we did together. They covered aspects such as hope, as he was a firm believer that by someone having hope in their life and a reason for living this would reduce the self-harm both in frequency and severity. How was I going to get from A (infertility due to endometriosis a significant factor in my self-harm) to B (a baby). I had another acute admission due to my depression and self-harm. I somehow had to cease self-harming long enough to be accepted as a paying IVF patient. This was incredibly hard for me, but the prospect of having a baby over-rode the desire to self-harm and I temporarily stopped.

Things did change significantly when I had children these years becoming some of the most stable I have had. I continued to be supported by the specialist self-harm nurse who understood the self-harm and didn't focus solely on the self-harm. I have also been fortunate to be registered with an excellent GP who has been supportive of my numerous hospital admissions and the self-harm. This GP has been my backbone at times. I have an appointment with him fortnightly (or weekly if he is very concerned). My GP describes my self-harm as a coping strategy, which it is. He prescribes sterile strips and dressings in order that I can manage my self-harm myself without Accident and Emergency attendance.

I became involved in the Better Services for people who Self Harm project, run by the Royal College of Psychiatrists. I was able to share my lived experience of self-harm locally to where I lived. By this point I had attended Accident and Emergency department many, many times. Sometimes I would be treated with dignity and compassion. All too often though, I was made to feel worthless. I recall being told, 'there are really poorly people here', the clear inference being I wasn't worthy of treatment or compassion. One of the worst elements was, being 'taught a lesson'. Unfortunately, some people who self-harm haven't always been offered pain relief when requiring suturing. Barbaric. One of the outcomes from the Better Services for people who Self Harm project was that staff in both Mental Health settings and the Accident and Emergency settings acknowledged that they had a poor understanding of self-harm and why people self-harm. I was asked to develop a teaching programme for the staff, which very much focused on the lived experience perspective. I recall, thinking I didn't have the skills to do such work and my confidence in my ability to do this being rock bottom. With support and encouragement, I was able to fulfil this role. This work continues to this day and is empowering for me. Only recently during an acute admission, two members of staff commented on attending the lecturers I deliver at a local University, and the positive impact it had on their practice.

One of the worst things that has happened to me during my journey was during an acute admission. At the time my local mental health provider would allow limited access to my razor blade. It was all care planned; I would be allowed 5–10 min-

utes with the blade on the condition that I self-harmed superficially. I had asked a nurse for access to my blade, and it was agreed that they would return in 10 minutes' time. I had the appropriate equipment to stem blood flow, sterile strips and sterile solution. After 10 minutes, I awaited the nurses return but they didn't. I was genuinely scared that if I continued to cut after the 10 minutes, I would be in trouble and may not be allowed my blade again. After over an hour I approached the nurse to remind them, they acknowledged me and said they would be there in a minute. However, this never materialised and instead I was left with my blade. By this time, I couldn't tolerate looking at it, such was the urge to do some significant damage. I hid the blade inside a drawer in an effort to avoid eye contact with it. My anxiety was gaining momentum. I lay on my bed in my room, scared that I would be the person who was blamed for still having access to their razor blade. After what felt like an eternity (though in reality was probably 3 hours) I left my room to try and find another member of staff. I found someone who I got on well with and requested they come to my room, where I blurted out about the razor blade and trying to get help. The member of staff understandably wanted to know how much damage I had done with having my blade for such a long length of time. Mercifully, the damage was limited, and I didn't require hospital attention. The lack of respect and care shown by this nurse will live with me forever. I appreciate and understand the care planning of being allowed a blade for a short period of time is a contentious topic, with many professionals not agreeing with it. However, in my opinion it is an area that needs to be discussed in an open and safe arena.

I have had genuinely scary times when I have bled heavily. One such time I attended Accident and Emergency and I knew I was bleeding heavily despite me trying to stem the blood flow. I was seen quickly by an auxiliary who informed me I would be triaged next. I waited and waited, and numerous other people were called into triage before me. After about 45–60 minutes I went to speak with reception and there were gasps of horror as the pool of blood became apparent. I was rushed through (no triage) and a bed trolley appeared and I was asked to get on it and taken to resus. It became clear how heavily I was bleeding and I felt faint due to the blood loss. The nurse was amazing, talking to me in a friendly way, reassuring me as he and the Doctor did what was necessary to stem the blood loss. Once this was more under control, there was then the conversation of whether surgery was appropriate. I was lucky, the Doctor was able to suture me, and he did so with compassion and care. When it came to my discharge, I sat up, the room began to spin and I felt very dizzy. More observations were carried out and a finger prick blood test taken. I remember the nurse being shocked at how low my blood count results were and said the machine must be wrong. A full blood count was organised, and I was severely anaemic. Staff were uncomfortable with me driving home so my partner was called to take me home.

The Accident and Emergency department can range from compassionate Doctors who spend time with you and ensure that you receive local anaesthetic before they suture. Such Doctors maintain appropriate eye contact, speak gently, and ensure that the tugging as they suture is not causing me pain. However, there is the other side of the coin the Doctors who cannot even look at you in the eye, speak to you in an uncaring way, describe the self-harm as 'attention seeking'. Only recently when I attended Accident & Emergency a nurse and two Doctors all agreed that I required suturing, only to be overruled by a colleague, who barely looked at the deep cut, nor me and said, 'don't bother suturing'. I was left with a gaping hole covered by a dressing over it. Fortunately, my support worker was able to utilise some of my sterile strips to close *the deep wound. My support worker strongly advised I attend Accident and Emergency, but I felt too humiliated.*

To conclude self-harm is a coping strategy and a way for me to manage overwhelming distress. Over 20 years later I am still on a journey of self-harm. I believe it will always play a part in my life. This saddens me. However, I have recently begun DBT (dialectical behaviour therapy) where the aim is to reduce the impulsivity of my self-harm. It is early days for this therapy... and all I can do for now is hope.

UNDERSTANDING SELF-HARM

Self-harm is defined as intentional self-poisoning or injury that is non-suicidal (National Institute for Health and Care Excellence [NICE], 2022; American Psychiatric Association [APA], 2013). The 2014 Adult Psychiatric Morbidity Survey in England shows that approximately 6.4% of adults (16 to 74 years old) report self-harming at some point in their lives. In 16- to 24-year-old women, this percentage is much higher, with 25.7% (1 in 4) reporting they have self-harmed (McManus et al., 2016). These figures represent a rise in reported self-harm compared to data from the previous decade, and the data is mirrored in Hospital Episode Data where some individuals attending hospital for treatment have identified self-harm as the method of injury. Self-harm can occur at any stage across the lifespan, and while it is non-suicidal, it can sometimes culminate into suicide whether accidentally or otherwise. Self-harm can be experienced across a range of physical and mental health conditions, although it is more strongly associated with the latter. Many individuals who self-harm struggle with intolerable distress or extremely difficult situations, and they might experience these difficulties for some time before they self-harm (Royal College of Psychiatrists, 2014). This resonates with Betty who describes her experiences of trauma and abuse from childhood and explains that self-harm through cutting herself and medication overdoses began much later, after the loss of her first pregnancy.

What is often challenging for family, friends and healthcare professionals is understanding why an individual might self-harm. While there might be many different reasons why, individuals with lived experience of self-harm report it is often a way to cope with difficult life circumstances such as loss, relationship difficulties and socio-economic hardships; and a way of relieving distressing or overwhelming feelings, anger, tension, anxiety and depression (Baker, 2017; McManus et al., 2016). Therefore, it is important to understand self-harm from Betty's perspective and experience. For the mental health nurse, a useful starting point for exploring self-harm and what underlies Betty's emotional distress is to engage in a collaborative assessment with Betty. This is likely to uncover the myriad of experiences that have contributed to how Betty might be feeling. In Fig. 7.1 we use the image of an iceberg which can aid our understanding by bringing into sharp focus Betty's cumulative experiences of abuse, trauma, loss, guilt, shame, embarrassment, emotional distress and how all this forms the strong base of an iceberg that is hidden below the water line. All we

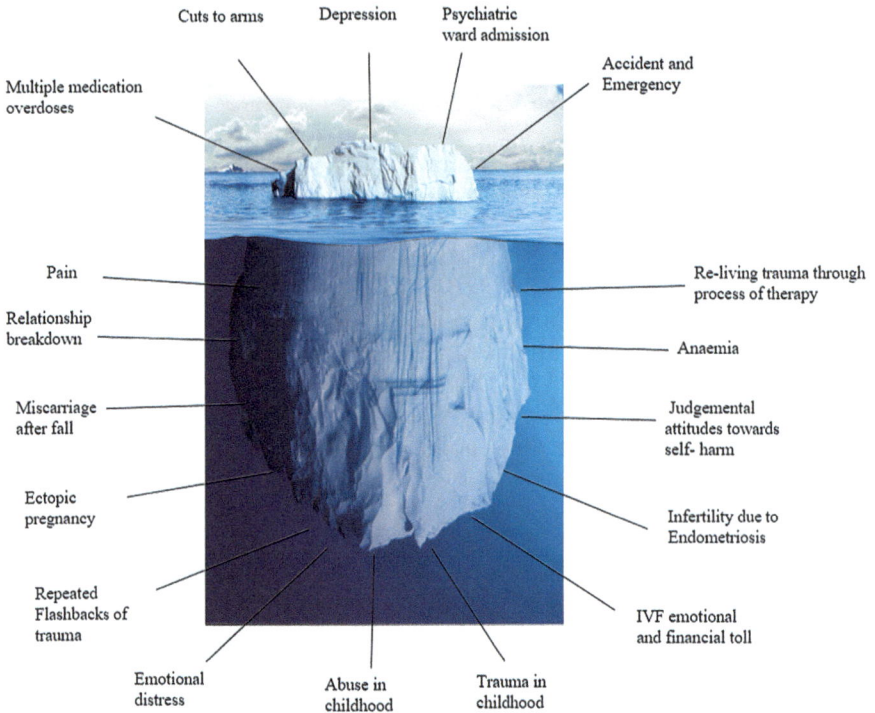

Fig. 7.1 Visualising Betty's experience of distress and self-harm through iceberg imagery. (Credit: Iceberg Image (without text) from Microsoft 365 Stock Images)

see is the 'tip' of the iceberg, which represents the external aspects of Betty accessing accident and emergency services and mental health services in crisis, and how she is coping and finding relief through self-harm and medication overdoses. A mental health nurse seeking to understand and help make sense of Betty's life events and experiences, would delve a little deeper towards the base of the iceberg, and explore these areas sensitively through assessment and formulation.

How a Mental Health Nurse Might Approach Assessment and Formulation: A Home Treatment Team Example

In this chapter, we provide an example of how Betty might be referred from Accident and Emergency (A&E) to a Home Treatment Team (HTT) as an alternative to a psychiatric hospital admission. Psychiatric hospital admissions can play an important part in minimising risk and enabling 24-hour assessment and care provision for an individual who may be experiencing severe emotional distress, self-harm or suicidal intent (Eunson et al., 2012). However, this does depend on a variety of factors. Data from a study that explored the treatment effect of hospitalisation for suicidal behaviour shows hospitalisation can reduce suicide risk immediately after a suicide attempt, but not for the year after that as hospitalisation actually increased the risks of suicide attempts (Ross et al., 2024). We know from the literature and from anecdotal evidence that hospitalisation can interrupt an individual's day-to-day normal routine and ward environments can also be very rigid—requiring an individual to follow certain rules and times that may not fit with routines they are accustomed to in their own home. This can be dis-empowering for an individual and may inadvertently reinforce feelings of hopelessness and helplessness. If a hospital admission is required, it would be important to consider discharge as a vulnerable point for an individual, therefore robust multidisciplinary planning would help ensure that the individual has a smoother transition back to their home environment. Conversely, if a HTT referral is appropriate for an individual, (in our example, appropriate for Betty), this may offer the least restrictive way of collaboratively exploring and supporting Betty to manage the wave of crisis with minimal interruption to her usual routine.

Formulation is a process that facilitates a deeper understanding of an individual's experiences of distress, and the surrounding circumstances, with a view to then exploring what might help reduce their emotional distress (Hartley, 2021). It is informed by information gathered at assessment, and it draws on a relevant theoretical framework to help with making sense of and explaining an individual's experiences (in context). Formulation does not necessarily aim to diagnose, although this depends on the model of working used by a professional. The HTT might take a biopsychosocial approach to formulation, beginning with a collaborative biopsychosocial assessment of Betty's lived experience using a standardised template that comprises of the headings in Table 7.1. Standardised assessments are often criticised for being too rigid and lacking the flexibility for a more individualised assessment. That said, the rationale for having standardised templates is to ensure that all individuals who access a service can have a comprehensive assessment that considers all the key aspects of their life and experiences and can ensure consistent application across all service users.

The information gathered in the assessment (Table 7.1) can enable mental health nurses in the HTT to begin collaboratively developing a formulation with Betty and enabling identification of her areas of need. What might not seem obvious from the standardised template is where the 'formulation' aspect happens. Arguably, the information in the standardised template can enable formulation, and a practitioner who is familiar with the process of formulation might work with this as it is. However, there are several formulation models which offer frameworks that can be helpful for facilitating the formulation process. Given that the HTT uses a biopsychosocial approach to assessment (and treatment), the main areas to explore for formulation could align with this and draw on theoretical explanatory frameworks—in this case the biopsychosocial model of health by Engel (1977). The Biopsychosocial Formulation would help in visualising the functional links between Betty's biological, psychological

Table 7.1   Standardised biopsychosocial assessment template

Reason for referral
Presenting complaint/situation
Teams involved
Triggers/Stressors
Past Psychiatric History and Psychological Treatments (psychiatric and psychological care history)
Medication
Personal History
Physical health
Social Circumstances
Allergies
Current support
Verbal consent to speak with relatives/carers/ friends
Mental Capacity Assessment
MENTAL STATE EXAMINATION:
Appearance/Behaviour
Speech
Mood
Sleep/Appetite
Thoughts
Cognition
Insight
Forensic History
Substance use—Alcohol/Drugs (Type, quantity, pattern, withdrawal & current help)
Risks
Safeguarding adults/children
Impression/summary
Plan

and social experiences with her current emotional distress and self-harm. Betty details a history of emotional distress that spans over 20 years, and with that comes a lot of information that would be recorded in her clinical notes. A formulation is beneficial in this instance as it would normally be on one A4 sheet of paper, serving as a summary and easy-to-visualise link between key aspects of Betty's experiences, her emotional distress and episodes of self-harm. An example of how an initial formulation might look like in practice is outlined in Table 7.2 below, and it summarises key information gathered from the biopsychosocial assessment and Betty's story:

The above represents an initial formulation using the information gathered so far, however there is scope for developing the formulation further through obtaining additional information, particularly where there are gaps in the assessment. Formulation is never fully complete, but it can develop and evolve as new information, experiences and circumstances emerge. A formulation can also continue to evolve after the treatment or interventions commence. The benefit of this is the opportunity for strengthening the therapeutic relationship and having a more responsive, targeted approach to intervention (Dudley & Kuyken, 2014). It is worth also noting that there is no right or

Table 7.2 Betty's initial biopsychosocial formulation

Biological: An initial formulation statement for the biological factors might be: Betty is a 42 year-old female. She has diagnoses of depression, anaemia and endometriosis. She has had a number of miscarriages and went through IVF to have children.

Psychological: Betty has attended A&E following an episode of self-harm through cutting her arms. She was experiencing a period of emotional distress prior to this. [*We do not have information on what event or trigger led to the most recent self-harm incident, however this can become a point for further exploration.*] An initial formulation statement for the psychological factors might be: Betty has a history of trauma and abuse from childhood. She has a current diagnosis of depression for which she is prescribed medication. When she is experiencing emotional distress, she self-harms to manage the distressing emotions

Social: An initial formulation statement for the social factors might be: Betty is a mother of 3 children and she lives with her partner. Betty has worked as a hairdresser, and she is making valuable contributions to developing and educating health and care workforce on self-harm, co-production and supporting trauma informed care.

wrong way to undertake formulation because there can be different ways to interpret an individual's circumstances and different formulations can be developed with the same individual (Crowe et al., 2008). The focus ideally should be on the validity of the formulation, establishing whether the explanatory and theoretical frameworks make sense given the individual's experiences and context, and more importantly, whether the formulation has led to appropriate interventions that have helped reduce the individual's emotional distress. With this in mind, Betty's formulation would not only hold in mind the information gathered during assessment, but it would also begin engaging with key theories that might help with making sense of her experiences. For example, she has experienced loss through miscarriages. Loss can trigger a range of difficult feelings such as grief, sadness, guilt and fear (Taylor & Shrive, 2023), therefore theory on loss might be helpful to explore with regard to how it might be impacting on Betty from the *biological, psychological* and *social* domains of the formulation. Other theories to explore could include theory on trauma and abuse. Betty has flashbacks of abuse and trauma from childhood. While flashbacks are a normal part of human experience (Taylor & Shrive, 2023), it would be important to recognise that Betty's flashbacks might be triggering her emotional distress as they force her to re-live the traumatic experiences of the past. This might explain how flashbacks may impact on her day-to-day life—and she manages the associated emotional distress through self-harm. Betty provides a vivid description of her experience of distress, using an analogy of a pressure cooker to illustrate how self-harm acts as the much needed release of the internal pressure and emotional distress she feels. The formulation should also recognise strengths and protective factors (Johnstone, 2018). The initial formulation of *social factors* in Table 7.2 makes an initial attempt at recognising and spotlighting her protective factors. Betty has lived with the trauma of abuse since childhood, and as such her feelings of being overwhelmed and emotionally distressed have persisted over a long time. Through it all, hers is a story of survival, perseverance despite the odds, and a testament to how she has held on with hope, particularly when she has interacted with mental health and general hospital staff who showed compassion and a genuine interest in understanding her distress.

PLANNING CARE BASED ON THE FORMULATION

Following assessment and biopsychosocial formulation with Betty, a plan of care would be developed using the HTT care planning template. Care plan templates receive similar criticisms in that there is a risk of them becoming a tick box exercise. This may be compounded by the environmental pressures within services where high caseloads and insufficient time/resource might lead to a rushed process of assessment and care planning. Formulation would be an additional step that triggers a more meaningful or considered approach to care planning as it requires collaboration with Betty and development of a shared understanding of her emotional distress. Formulation therefore can provide a stronger basis for recommended interventions in the care plan. The care plan process would also prompt the exploration of how the HTT can support Betty to reduce self-harm and explore alternative coping strategies while managing and reducing the emotional distress that underlies the self-harm.

The care plan template includes questions that would be central to this process being more collaborative—done 'with' Betty rather than 'to' her. For example, questions such as *What does recovery mean to you? What are your long-term goals and what do you want to achieve in the next year? What matters to you? What important things in your life might support your recovery? What skills, strengths and experiences will help you achieve your goals?* The mental health nurse would also ask Betty to rate the following items (Table 7.3) using Dialogue Plus which is a tool used in some UK National Health Service Trusts. The items are presented as a Likert Scale to measure how satisfied an individual is with the various areas of their life and health, and these areas would be considered when planning Betty's care.

Table 7.3   Likert Scale on satisfaction

Using the scale below (from 1 to 7) how would you rate the following:
1. Totally dissatisfied 2. Very dissatisfied 3. Fairly dissatisfied 4. In the middle 5. Fairly satisfied 6. Very satisfied 7. Totally satisfied
How satisfied are you with your mental health?
How satisfied are you with your physical health?
How satisfied are you with your job situation?
How satisfied are you with your accommodation?
How satisfied are you with your leisure activities?
How satisfied are you with your relationship with your partner/family?
How satisfied are you with your friendships?
How satisfied are you with your personal safety?
How satisfied are you with your medication?
How satisfied are you with the practical help you receive?
How satisfied are you with your meetings with mental health professionals?

In terms of interventions or treatment, the HTT team offers a variety of therapeutic interventions such as Mindfulness, Distress Tolerance Techniques, Solution Focussed Therapy and Open Dialogue. Where the formulation indicates strength in a particular therapeutic approach this could be delivered within the HTT. If a therapeutic treatment is not available within the HTT staff resource, a referral to an additional service such as Improving Access to Psychological Therapies (IAPT) would be recommended. For Betty, this might be a service where she can access Dialectical Behaviour Therapy (DBT). DBT is 'an evidence based therapy aimed at helping individuals regulate their emotions through developing an awareness of different emotional states and learning ways to cope with these'. It is often recommended for individuals who may use coping strategies such as self-harm, and it offers tools and techniques for recognition of early warning signs and changes to an individual's emotional or cognitive state that they can then work on regulating (Augustus et al., 2019).

Betty outlines a previous care plan that included an agreement for her to have razors for 10 minutes and make superficial cuts, then access to sterile strips for wound management. Harm minimisation approaches can minimise chances of infection and severe scarring or excessive bleeding (Baker, 2017). Betty recognises the contentious nature of the harm minimisation approach, and her sentiments are echoed in the literature around harm minimisation approaches more broadly with the debates centring around whether approaches such as needle exchange programmes, or access to razors for self-harm should be offered or not. One study that explored prevalence, socio-demographic and clinical characteristics of individuals who self-harm and use harm minimisation strategies, found that a small number of patients used harm minimisation interventions, and they found this very helpful for them (Cliffe et al., 2021). Betty describes being told by one nurse to 'just stop it'. This can be an unhelpful way of approaching self-harm because it risks minimising the reality of [the individuals] experiences and possibly distressing emotions and does not open the door towards effective therapeutic working (Baker, 2017, pp. 312–313). Furthermore, due consideration would need to be given to what supportive alternatives can be put in place first for an individual manage their overwhelming feelings and emotional distress. During formulation, this would be explored sensitively, with holistic and multidisciplinary discussion that also considers risk and safety for Betty. Engendering hope and a non-judgemental approach would be an important part of supporting Betty, as she identified in her story that the mental health professionals who were compassionate and worked in a hope filled way made a real difference to her experience and recovery. This is crucial given the stigma associated with self-harm. It is helpful for the mental health nurse to look beyond the self-harm and see the individual. Self-harm makes up only one small element of an individual's life—as they may be a mother, daughter, son, father, partner, with interests, hobbies, jobs, and other aspects about them that could be focussed upon to embrace a strengths-based approach (Anderson & Waters, 2009; Baker, 2017). There is an increase in literature that amplifies voices of individuals with lived experience and the valuable contributions that they can and do make, and this needs to be acknowledged (O'Brien & Davenport, 2024).

A mental health nurse may consider the CHIME conceptual framework for personal recovery from mental illness which outlines 5 key components of Connectedness, Hope and Optimism about the future, Identity, Meaning in life and Empowerment which would be a helpful approach to supporting Betty (Leamy et al., 2011; Bird et al., 2014).

In summary, there are different ways of supporting individuals who are experiencing emotional distress with associated self-harm. This chapter provided one example of how a HTT may approach assessment formulation and care planning in collaboration with Betty. The HTT gives insight into a model of care and support that would prioritise formulation and interventions in the individuals home environment. There is scope for mental health nurses to leverage their role in the different settings they work in to explore ways of integrating (or recognising) where a formulation approach might provide a bridge between assessment and interventions and prioritise person-centred collaboration with the individual who is struggling with their mental health and self-harm. There is increased recognition of the role and importance of Trauma Informed Care, and training to support greater understanding of how trauma may impact on mental health (Gerber, 2019). Trauma informed care is based on an understanding of and responsiveness to trauma—emphasizing physical, psychological and emotional safety for both services and individuals who are struggling with their mental health (Substance Abuse and Mental Health Services Administration [SAMHSA], 2014). Betty identifies in her story that there is scope for mental health nurses (and healthcare professionals more broadly) to have a better understanding of self-harm, and knowledge of supportive ways to work with individuals who may self-harm. Trauma informed care also contributes towards reducing some of the stigma and judgmental attitudes in healthcare. It fosters a more compassionate approach to supporting individuals through considering the role that trauma may have played in their lives, and how they have adapted to manage in the circumstances.

Points for Reflection
1. Reflect on what your thoughts are about self-harm? Consider what fears, views or uncertainties you have about self-harm.
2. After reading this chapter, how might you approach an individual who is experiencing emotional distress and self-harming to try and cope with the distress? Think about what you might say, or what resources you might draw on to develop your understanding of self-harm.
3. Explore a few service user led resources about self-harm (for example through https://www.madinamerica.com/), and make note of whether you notice any similarities or differences in perspectives and management of self-harm when compared to national guidelines and resources (for example through https://www.nice.org.uk/)

REFERENCES

American Psychiatric Association. (2013). *Diagnostic and statistical manual of mental disorders* (5th ed.). American Psychiatric Association Publishing. Retrieved March 13, 2024, from https://www.appi.org/dsm

Anderson, M., & Waters, K. (2009). Recognition and therapeutic management of self-harm and suicidal behaviour, Chapter 17. In P. Callaghan, J. Playle, & L. Copper (Eds.), *Mental health nursing skills*. Oxford University Press.

Augustus, J., Williams, B., & Bold, J. (2019). *Interventions*. In J. Augustus, B. Williams, & J. Bold (Eds.), *An introduction to mental health*. Sage.

Baker, C. (2017). *Working with self-harm and suicide*. In A. Clifton, S. Hemmingway, A. Felton, & G. Stacey (Eds.), *Fundamentals of mental health nursing: An essential guide for nursing and healthcare students* (1st ed.). John Wiley and Sons.

Bird, V., Leamy, M., Tew, J., Le Boutillier, C., Williams, J., & Slade, M. (2014). Fit for purpose? Validation of a conceptual framework for personal recovery with current mental health consumers. *Australian & New Zealand Journal of Psychiatry, 48*(7), 644–653. https://doi.org/10.1177/0004867413520046

Cliffe, C., Pitman, A., Sedgwick, R., Pritchard, M., Dutta, R., & Rowe, S. (2021). Harm minimisation for the management of self-harm: A mixed-methods analysis of electronic health records in secondary mental healthcare. *BJPsych Open, 7*(4), e116. https://doi.org/10.1192/bjo.2021.946

Crowe, M., Carlyle, D., & Farmer, R. (2008). Clinical formulation for mental health nursing practice. *Journal of Psychiatric and Mental Health Nursing, 15*, 800–807.

Dudley, R., & Kuyken, W. (2014). Case formulation in cognitive behavioural therapy, chapter 2. In L. Johnstone & R. Dallos (eds.), *Formulation in psychology and psychotherapy: Making sense of peoples problems* (2nd ed.). Routledge.

Engel, G. L. (1977). The need for a new medical model: A challenge for biomedicine. *Science, 196*(4286), 129–136. https://doi.org/10.1126/science.847460

Eunson, H., Grout, G., Pritchard, J., & Carthy, J. (2012). Developing nursing decision making skills, Chapter 7. In S. Tee, J. Brown, & D. Carpenter (Eds.), *Handbook of mental health nursing*. Hodder Arnold.

Gerber, M. (2019). *Trauma informed healthcare approaches: A guide for primary care*. Springer.

Hartley, S. (2021). Using team formulation in mental health practice. *Mental Health Practice*. https://doi.org/10.7748/mhp.2021.e1516

Johnstone, L. (2018). Psychological formulation as an alternative to psychiatric diagnosis. *Journal of Humanistic Psychology, 58*(1), 30–46. https://doi.org/10.1177/0022167817722230

Leamy, M., Bird, V., Le Boutillier, C., Williams, J., & Slade, M. (2011). Conceptual framework for personal recovery in mental health: Systematic review and narrative synthesis. *The British Journal of Psychiatry: The Journal of Mental Science, 199*(6), 445–452. https://doi.org/10.1192/bjp.bp.110.083733

McManus, S., Bebbington, P., Jenkins, R., & Brugha, T. (Eds.). (2016). *Mental health and wellbeing in England: Adult psychiatric morbidity survey 2014*. NHS Digital.

National Institute for Health and Care Excellence (2022) *Self-harm: Assessment, management and preventing recurrence* NG225. National Institute for Health and Care Excellence

O'Brien, S., & Davenport, C. (2024). Embedding the service user voice to co-produce UK mental health nurse education. A lived experience narrative. *Journal of Psychiatric and Mental Health Nursing, 00*, 1–7. https://doi.org/10.1111/jpm.13031

Ross, E. L., Bossarte, R. M., Dobscha, S. K., et al. (2024). Estimated average treatment effect of psychiatric hospitalization in patients with suicidal behaviors: A precision treatment analysis. *JAMA Psychiatry, 81*(2), 135–143. https://doi.org/10.1001/jamapsychiatry.2023.3994

Royal College of Psychiatrists. (2014). Self-harm. Retrieved January 21, 2024, from www.rcpsych.ac.uk/healthadvice/problemsdisorders/self-harm.aspx

Substance Abuse and Mental Health Services Administration [SAMHSA] (2014). *SAMHSA's concept of trauma and guidance for a trauma-informed approach.* HHS Publication No. (SMA) 14-4884. Substance Abuse and Mental Health Services Administration.

Taylor, J., & Shrive, J. (2023). *Indicative trauma impact manual.* Victim Focus.

CHAPTER 8

Practitioner Reflections on the Use of Formulation in Mental Health Nursing Practice

Vickie Howard, Jane Peirson, Michelle Gideon, and Michelle Martin

Key Learning Points
- Accounts of mental health nurses' and other professionals' experiences of using formulation
- Mental health nursing contexts of using formulation
- A discussion summary of themes
- Indications for future exploration, development and research

Contributors: Toby Bell, Gemma Boswell, Jade Graves, Rachel Ramsbottom, Pamela Johnson, Eren Mills, Courtney Lamb, Lizzie Richardson, Jeanette Jones-Bragg, Lynette Robinson, Emma Ballantyne, Bridget Flynn, Natalie Turner.

V. Howard (✉)
Faculty of Health Sciences, University of Hull, Hull, UK
e-mail: V.Howard@Hull.ac.uk

J. Peirson
York St John University, York, UK
e-mail: j.peirson@yorksj.ac.uk

M. Gideon
East London Foundation Trust, London, UK
e-mail: gidds29@gmail.com

M. Martin
Faculty of Health Sciences, University of Hull, Hull, UK
e-mail: Michelle.Martin@Hull.ac.uk

© The Author(s), under exclusive license to Springer Nature Switzerland AG 2024
V. Howard, L. Alfred (eds.), *Formulation in Mental Health Nursing*,
https://doi.org/10.1007/978-3-031-59956-9_8

161

Introduction

This chapter will present and examine mental health care professionals' involvement in formulation and views focused on mental health nurses' roles and involvement in formulation practice. Beginning with student mental health nurses' excerpts from three students' reflections concerning using formulation, specific learning and areas of consideration will be highlighted.

The remainder of the chapter will present discursive reflections and practitioner accounts from registered mental health nurses and other mental health professionals on areas of formulation practice. Key issues which have come to light will be thematically presented and discussed in the conclusion of this chapter, with regard to what these may indicate for continuing future formulation practice and research.

Student Mental Health Nurses' Formulation Reflections

Toby Bell: Themes—Understanding Formulation, Theory to Practice

Throughout the learning process and the process of formulation, I felt mostly confused. Formulation is something I had been involved in when out on placement, however I had not fully understood the process and I was not so familiar with the theory behind formulation. The confusion arose when the literature explained there was no clear definition or singular approach to formulation (Geach et al., 2017). Because of this, I struggled with gaining an initial understanding of the topic. There were some positives and negatives to the process of formulation and my learning. One of the positives I gained from carrying out the formulation is that I developed a deeper level of understanding of John's situation (the client I was working with). This helped in understanding John's problems beyond his diagnosis (Johnstone, 2018). I became more familiar with the 5Ps approach to formulation and would feel more confident in applying this in the future. One negative I took from carrying out the formulation is how little I initially knew about the procedure, however, upon further reading and researching, I saw my knowledge grow. Upon analysing the situation, it was understandable to feel confused when being introduced to a new way of working. This situation has provided a good opportunity to learn and develop a key skill needed for a registered nurse, as the skills involved in formulation correspond largely with The Code's requirements (Cox, 2020). To conclude this reflection, I believe the overall process of formulation was successful, and I now understand the application of the theory to practice in the real world. Lucy Johnstone's significant contribution to the body of research has helped develop my understanding, allowing me to form my own perspective on formulation. Moving forward, I would like to explore different approaches to formulation such as the psychodynamic approach. Doing this would give me the ability to have a broader knowledge of formulation and I would also be able to choose the approach I feel appropriate. This would allow me to adopt different approaches dependent on the needs of the individual and this would facilitate person-centred care, as per The Code (NMC, 2018).

Gemma Boswell: Themes—Formulation Use and Dementia, the Therapeutic Relationship

Formulation is considered a beneficial method within mental health nursing, as when the process is followed correctly, it can assist the practitioner to develop an understanding of the issues affecting the individual and why they are occurring, thus creating a foundation for appropriate intervention (Hartley, 2021). Furthermore, having been largely accepted for over 30 years as a key principle within clinical practice, formulation is a key component within the assessment and intervention process, which generally occurs as part of multidisciplinary approaches to the patient and practitioner therapeutic alliance (Baird et al., 2017). Due to the complexities of Jean's (service user I worked with) presenting cognitive disturbances combined with recurring anxiety and depression, the behaviours that challenge (BtC) formulation as a process (see: British Psychological Society's Dementia Advisory Group, 2018; Surrey Place, 2024) could be adopted, incorporating the multidisciplinary team (MDT) and following a systematic chain; acronym HELP; Health, Environment, Life Experience and Psychiatric conditions.

However further research argues that formulation is often delayed and even dismissed within both community and care facilities, due to the lack of education, and the misinterpretation of its meaning (McKenna et al., 2022). Although the BtC formulation could be presented as a formulation to consider as a pathway for Jean, it could be argued, that due to Jean's recurring presentation of anxiety and depression, cognitive behavioural therapy (CBT) may prove beneficial. Spector et al. (2012) explain many dementia sufferers do display such symptoms, which often manifest as increased agitation and aggression, therefore, a case formulation of the 5Ps (Presenting, Precipitating, Perpetuating, Predisposing and Protective factors) could be considered. Nevertheless, the practitioner should be aware of Jean's level of functioning, and ability to engage in CBT, with experts advising such therapies should commence as early as possible, stating ideally, the issue would be recognised before any cognitive impairment takes form (Stott, 2018). Having considered the different approaches to formulation, the most appropriate pathway for Jean, which will incorporate her current needs, yet address her past issues which present as anxiety and depression, would be the BtC formulation, as studies suggest this approach can provide practitioners with a greater perception of "stress and distress" (James & Reichelt, 2019). Within this model, Engel's biopsychosocial framework can be incorporated, giving the practitioner a broader understanding of Jean's needs, and aiding the establishment of a meaningful therapeutic relationship

(McKenzie & Brown, 2020). However, it is beneficial in the formulation for Jean, to consider Kitwood's personhood model, which has been developed specifically for the care and treatment of individuals with dementia. It focuses on six psychological needs (love, comfort, identity, occupation, inclusion and attachment) (Kaufmann & Engel, 2014).

Studies suggest that development of a significant therapeutic relationship and involving Jean in her care will rely heavily upon the practitioner's knowledge, understanding and empathetic approach to her biopsychosocial needs, and any previous traumatic life events which are proven in 70% of patients to contribute to the development of dementia (Wang et al., 2016). Furthermore, Peplau's interpersonal framework for psychodynamic nursing informs the practitioner of the importance of engaging in a collaboration with the patient for a successful alliance to be established (Deane & Fain, 2015). However, Nyström (2007) argues that the psychodynamic framework alone may prove unfruitful in the development of the nurse-patient relationship, adding that Peplau's theory should be utilised alongside discussing the existential issues Jean may be encountering and could be affecting her current presentations.

NICE guidelines (2018) indicate that where workable, it is imperative to involve the patient with a diagnosis of dementia as much as possible in their care formulation, modifying methods of communication utilising simplified texts and visual aids wherever necessary, and providing Jean and her immediate care network the relevant information relating to her condition. Furthermore, outstanding provision for post diagnosis support has been streamed in certain parts of the UK, however this is not available in all areas, with funding relying on a postcode lottery. Although this is not the result of the practitioners involved in Jean's care, and by no means reflects their capabilities, unfortunately, the therapeutic relationship and involvement of Jean and her family in the formulation could be negatively affected by the lack of area funding, a prospect which has been highlighted in the Prime Minister's challenge on dementia (GOV UK, 2022). Furthermore, Livingston et al., (2022) highlight the importance of recognising the physical illnesses the patient may encounter and provide post diagnostic support to prevent avoidable hospitalisations which could trigger agitation and aggression in patients such as Jean.

It is suggested that the involvement of Jean and her family in the BtC formulation process will impact positively upon the nurse-patient therapeutic relationship, as studies highlight the more informed the individual, there is a decrease in feelings of unease when interventions take place. Furthermore, the family members may adopt key skills in the management of escalating behaviours (Holle et al., 2017). However, the practitioner must be mindful of the cognitive capabilities of Jean, and her understanding of the formulation process (Stott, 2018).

The practitioner should be mindful, when constructing the BtC formulation with Jean of the Mental Capacity Act (2005) and its guidance, which is designed to protect the rights of people lacking the capacity to make informed decisions regarding their overall welfare (NICE, 2018). However, historically, emphasis has been placed on studies surrounding medical models of assessment, and therefore evidence relevant to the effects on the human rights of the individual may possibly be inadequate (Boyle, 2008).

Jade Graves: Themes—Team Formulation, Client Involvement

Christofides et al. (2012) found team formulations to be beneficial for the majority; however, they discovered this was the case within teams that fully understood the purpose of team formulation. Psychiatric teams who did not have a clearly defined role of formulation appeared to have greater barriers. Tinemakomboreroashe (2015) discovered team formulation within community settings provided professionals with a broader understanding of service users, an opportunity to gather information to explore any previous interventions, history and trauma. This also provides opportunity for shared exploration of ideas, risk management and staff validation. Following a systematic review conducted by Geach et al. (2017), findings show positive results and lie in agreement with Christofides et al. (2012) and Tinemakomboreroashe (2015), however, research in this domain lacks enough evidence for a definite explanation. Sam's (person supported) formulation will be conducted through a team formulation, this has been decided due to the distress Sam experiences when discussing past events and another deciding factor was due to the difficulty of leaving her own home. Conducting a formulation with Sam in her own home would potentially leave Sam alone within her safe space with the past trauma and this would not be beneficial, Sam agreed with this.

As a care co-ordinator, it is important to explain the process and keep Sam updated so she feels involved as much as possible. A holistic assessment and formulation were conducted to assess, plan, implement and evaluate Sam's care (Lloyd, 2010). This looked at the most relevant evidenced-based research to enable the use of effective approaches and models, looking at the importance of therapeutic relationships and barriers which may occur. Although Sam was not a participant in the formulation, I believe it is important to inform her of the process to ensure she agreed with the team formulation method. Following the formulation, Sam may wish to revisit or understand what interventions will be put in place. I explained to Sam we would look at the implications together to ensure she would be fully involved in the decision-making process and was able to make informed choices. Being honest, supportive, compassionate and, empathetic allowed trust to be built, this has been a major contribution in maintaining the therapeutic relationship. I feel strongly about keeping Sam informed but also must ensure I always consider what is best for the individual. To improve, it will be beneficial to participate in an individual formulation and to further understand the theory. It is imperative to decide the formulation technique for each individual and to be as inclusive as possible, considering their wishes, beliefs and values. It is important to understand an individual may benefit from participating in the formulation process, but to also consider the distress this may cause by re-experiencing past events. To achieve this, I will continue to contribute to assessments and formulations and assess, discuss and decide the best option going forward. I aim to do this within the final year in placements and going forward as a newly qualified nurse.

Registered Mental Health Nurses' and Other Professionals' Views on Formulation and How This Fits with Current Practice and Roles

Rachel Ramsbottom—Senior Practitioner/Community Mental Health Nurse in Adult Mental Health (Early Intervention in Psychosis Service)

A bit about me—I have been qualified as a MHN (mental health nurse) since 2005 and have experience of working in several different early intervention teams as well as in a post as a Psychosocial Interventions Practitioner in a CMHT (community mental health team). I have been working in my current team for 14 years and have progressed to a senior practitioner role. I am currently undertaking a Postgraduate Diploma in Advanced Mental Health Practice which qualifies you to apply for warranting as an Approved Mental Health Practitioner (AMHP). There is a further part of the programme which leads to obtaining an MA degree. The course is open to individuals from different professional backgrounds, though nurses are hugely underrepresented within the AMHP field.

My thoughts about formulation—through my career I have learnt and have applied experience of using various types of formulation (CBT for psychosis, Stress vulnerability model, 5Ps and the power threat meaning framework).

As a care co-ordinator early on in my career, I had the opportunity to access training and supervision from psychology to develop formulations that helped me understand and make sense of people's distress beyond the illness model. I am very passionate about understanding people's experiences in the context of their life experiences and developing a collaborative understanding to support people on their journey.

My skills and experiences of formulation were further developed and enhanced during my two-year role as a Psychosocial Interventions Practitioner. This post was split into both a care co-ordinator role and psychosocial interventions (PSI) practitioner role. I think my experience of using formulation within this role was more intensive. Formulation was essential to the assessment process and informed the chosen interventions. I was delivering CBTP (cognitive behavioural therapy for psychosis) and family interventions under high levels of supervision and had access to some excellent training in CBTP. In each community team there was at least one or two PSI practitioners from any professional background. For the PSI work, we receive high levels of supervision from the psychologists and high levels of training and we delivered CBTP informed interventions. It was a really interesting role. Inhouse training was available and there was a lot of CPD (continuing professional development) and a lot of learning on the job. We delivered CBTP informed therapy specifically to individuals under the CMHT with psychosis, schizophrenia and bipolar.

The challenges I have had in the past was when my role was split; it was difficult having a therapy caseload (15) as well as a care co-ordinator caseload (7). It was quite challenging to manage. I had some complex cases under the CMHT that required safeguarding and crisis work and I was also running a weekly group. I was learning on the job, offering CBTP-based interventions and family work and then with the care co-ordinator work—I felt I was being pulled in so many directions and found it hard to consolidate the learning at the same time and being a perfectionist didn't help!

In the end I went back to the care co-ordinator role in EIS (Early Interventions Service) because I found it too hard being pulled in different directions. Interestingly, in some of the other boroughs, the PSI practitioners didn't also have the care co-ordination caseload which I think can be challenging when you are trying to provide consistency and you are newer to developing therapy skills.

The context of my current role now—I almost don't feel like a nurse! By that I mean I feel set back from nursing. I've been working in the same early intervention team for around 14 years now but more recently I have progressed to senior practitioner role within the team. So, I'm kind of split between holding a small complex caseload and undertaking management and leadership tasks including supervision and clinical leadership etc.

Within my EIS post over the years I have found that whilst we have used a range of formulations as part of the assessment process, it remains a challenge in terms of time, space, support and ongoing supervision.

When I compare the space I used to have in comparison to what I have now and what nurses and allied professionals have now coming into community posts, time constraints are a huge and significant barrier to being able to do the PSI therapeutic work.

My use of formulation—The main models of formulation I am familiar with is the 5Ps, the power threat meaning framework and CBT formulation. In trying to work towards being more trauma informed we are looking at our eight-week assessment pathway and considering how we can improve things and bringing back formulations during the assessment period was felt to be really important. Ensuring an opportunity to think more psychologically about a person's distress is essential.

The opportunity, learning and space to undertake formulation can be challenging within the team as it is currently due to the increasing pressures and social care demands. It almost feels like now the service is more focused on trying to firefight and address the significant social care issues. I find myself and the care co-ordinators wanting to do this important and meaningful work but again finding ourselves being pulled in so many directions…so there's trying to manage all the crisis, the housing and the financial kind of stuff. But then there's also trying to meet the KPIs (key performance indicators). I think if I reflect on the amount of time I spend these days on the computer rather than seeing people, it's crazy!

We are lucky to have an excellent psychology team who are so supportive, highly skilled and keen to support us in formulating and undertaking PSI interventions, and we have access to group supervision for complex case discussions where various formulation models are used such as the Power Threat Meaning Framework, which I really like. I have also used the hot cross bun—CBT but more informally as a Care Co-ordinator.

I have to admit I don't use formulation as much as I used to which I think is a real shame and I also see other nursing colleagues and students who have had very little opportunity to learn, develop and access training around formulation. My recent nursing students had never encountered formulation on their course teaching.

Formulation is always there in my mind when working with someone, but I just think there are a lot of barriers as people just don't have the time to do it which is a real shame. It is important and even doing the AMHP course—the reliance on the work and interventions done in the community is huge. It is important to undertake the preventative and recovery work in a least restrictive way which can have a significant impact on preventing detentions. Some people are going round and round in the system and it's not about the person—it's about system failure. Something in our system is not working! When will people acknowledge this?? You can observe it, the more stretched we are, the more risk averse and reactive we are rather than engaging in the proactive work that keeps people out of hospital. It's really tough as you cannot be proactive, implement assertive outreach and be creative and have space to develop the skills in PSI if you are constantly under pressure, burning out and firefighting. I also think the heavy focus on management aspects of supervision and not having a dedicated and regular clinical supervision space with someone skilled in PSI also contributes to these challenges. Whilst psychology offers the space, this is different to having dedicated supervision which is something in my previous teams I have really benefitted from.

I also believe leadership is absolutely essential, being able to model, prioritise, encourage, nurture your team, share the philosophy and vision and importance of formulation and PSI in promoting recovery within a service. This becomes the standard and expectation. There needs to be more space to allow nurses and allied professionals to do the psychologically informed work that can have such a powerful impact on recovery. As an early interventions service, relapse prevention work is key, however more recently it has not been a priority because of the high demand on care co-ordination responsibilities. One approach that I have found really powerful in supporting recovery is the "Open Dialogue" approach. We have had a small pilot with some incredibly positive outcomes. Formulation of the distress and difficulties may be talked through together within the network meetings.

I want to take the opportunity to thank the professionals and service users / networks whom I have had the privilege to work with over the span of my career, have believed in me, I have learnt from, supported me, encouraged and developed me, offered me a safe space for clinical supervision and helped me thrive and become the practitioner that I am today.

Pamela Johnson—Mental Health Nurse Working in Older Adult Services (Memory Clinic)

What is formulation?—My understanding of using formulation involves professionals discussing a case based upon the needs and wishes of the patient. They will then formulate a plan to help address the individual's needs. My experience is based upon a multidisciplinary team approach involving doctors, nurses, psychologists, health care assistants and occupational therapists being involved in formulation.

The rationale behind formulation—We formulate to aid the diagnostic process but don't use a specific model. We also don't use formulation for every patient we see. Once information is gathered, the case is discussed with a medic who will formulate a diagnosis and treatment plan. There are times we will formulate when someone with dementia returns to our team for a review. This can be due to several reasons: carer stress, medication review, BPSD (behavioural and psychological symptoms in dementia).

The mental health nurse's role in formulation—Nurses tend to gather the information and usually lead the formulation meetings. Patients and carers are involved in formulation by collating their needs and wishes, which are incorporated into the formulation discussions.

Eren Mills: Mental Health Nurse—Team Leader at a Clinical Decisions Unit

My role—I am a band 7 Team Leader of a 14 bedded clinical decisions unit of mixed gender. The client group includes individuals with differing mental health diagnoses. On average the length of stay is three–five days, and we aim to assess people's mental health and signpost for support either in the community or further inpatient support and treatment.

My understanding of formulation—Formulation is a discussion to ascertain a person's circumstances, experiences and difficulties. This establishes how we can help and what the person may need and why.

My involvement in formulation—Nursing staff undertake one-to-one sessions alongside the psychologist. As part of the admission, we additionally complete a safety plan with patients and ask them questions around the 5Ps approach. This involves questions on their presenting problem and then predisposing factors, precipitating factors, perpetuating factors and protective factors. The service user is involved in co-completing the safety plan as part of the initial one-to-one meeting. They are offered a copy of their safety plan and requested to sign it.

What would help in developing formulation practice—I think it would help staff to understand their role in formulation, as it is often completed by a psychologist. I don't consider the work nursing staff do is recognised enough in how this adds to the formulation of a person, especially the information from the admission process and safety plan.

Lizzie Richardson—Lecturer in Mental Health, Previously Worked Five Years in the Access Team Which Was Previously Known as Single Point of Access (SPA)

I have experience of working within a community mental health team and within a number of inpatient mental health settings. I see formulation as a way of collating information and understanding someone's presentation to help guide the best course of treatment. With regard to training in formulation, I believe I had just one session many years ago in the NHS.

With regard to who is involved in formulation I consider this would be the patient, loved one if appropriate—though this can vary depending on the circumstances. I have been involved in formulation in the past through my role in access whereby nearly every assessment ended with a 5Ps formulation. The trust I worked for adapted their risk assessment to include a formulation approach which should have been updated each time the risk assessment was. In this service, the mental health nurse took a lead in the formulation, however with complex cases the formulation would be taken to the MDT and would be discussed in the psychological team. I consider that ideally the patient should be fully involved in the formulation. However, it was not uncommon for the patient to decline the invitation due to discussing past events being too difficult.

Courtney Lamb—Apprenticeship BSc Student Mental Health Nurse

I am a student nurse in year 3 working in a rehabilitation and recovery service for adults with mental health difficulties.

I understand formulations as creating a wider picture of the person's behaviours, characteristics, challenges and life experiences. This can then be put together to help develop an understanding of the person holistically which can assist in informing care and treatment planning.

In my working environment, we do formulations both individually as the nurse or key worker but also have set protected time to engage in group formulations with the whole team invited. This is made up of social workers, psychologists, nurses, support workers, occupational therapists and peer support workers. In the patients' safety plans we use the 5Ps. In the group formulation sessions, the psychologists lead this and we again use the 5Ps model.

Mental health nurses are involved in formulation as there is a section on the safety plan which uses the 5Ps model and this needs to be completed with the patient. In my service area, the nurses are responsible for completing the 5Ps for the group formulation sessions led by psychologists but using an MDT approach.

The service user is involved in the safety planning formulation in 1:1 time using the 5Ps model, however in the group formulation meetings the service user is not invited.

We studied a module on assessment and formulation at university in my apprenticeship undergraduate programme, however I do think in-service there should be more training around formulation. Sometimes I see formulations not being filled out or the offered timeslot for formulation is not always used which is a shame. I think formulation is an equal role for everyone involved in the patient's care however some nurses may feel as though it is more the part of a psychologist's job role.

Michelle Gideon—Mental Health Practitioner Working Across Primary and Secondary Care

The process of formulation attempts to homogenise large numbers of biopsychosocial causative factors which may lead to a deeper understanding of the service user's distress (Johnstone & Dallos, 2006).

"...But what does the patient want...?"

This simple question was one that I was ill equipped to answer to or advocate for when I first qualified as a mental health nurse in 2004.

Back then and from my experience, it really wasn't about what the patient wanted, but what the consultant decided was best because the psychiatrist was considered: All Powerful.

Nurses and junior doctors alike would often sit in silence, speaking only when spoken to, hastily scribbling notes and handing over medication cards for The Signature.

Diagnostic overshadowing (a practice by which health care professionals make assumptions about a person's behaviour based on their diagnosis) was commonplace because clinical discussions were often pre-occupied with the biological factors, so case formulation leaned predominantly towards the management of the biological symptoms of illness and of course, risk.

What I failed to realise then but seems glaringly obvious now, was that the service user was not at the centre of their treatment and their journeys were not really being heard or understood. By reducing the service users to just a handful of biological symptoms we, as mental health professionals, were potentially reinforcing a harmful, reductionist narrative that offered very little hope for their future.

Over time, there have been notable attempts to modernise the model in which mental health care, treatment and support is delivered to patients specifically within the community.

This current, transformative approach is centred around the Community Mental Health Framework which outlines NHS England's Long-Term Plan

(NHS England, 2017) for "Place-based community mental health" which is flexible and focuses on the whole person/whole population (NCCMH, 2021).

Nearly 20 years after qualifying, the most asked question within my daily multidisciplinary team huddle is: "…But what does the patient want?"

Only now, the psychiatrist sits alongside other clinical and non-clinical professionals from across community health and social care who have come together to cultivate a shared understanding of the patient's difficulties. I would suggest that perhaps informally, components of case/team formulation are becoming more widely embedded across primary and secondary care as more evidence-based, systematic approaches are being drawn upon to address the individual needs of each patient.

Formulation within these early stages, however, is more a process of communication between service providers in the form of written referrals. GPs write to the NMHT (Neighbourhood Mental Health Team) to request mental health input and will identify a starting point contextualised by the patient's biopsychosocial issues as well as the presenting problem, predisposing, precipitating, perpetuating and protective factors—also known as the 5Ps of formulation (Macneil et al., 2012).

Once the referral is screened by a senior triage nurse, formulation could be viewed as an event, as a prescribed set of actions will be implemented. An acknowledgement of the GP's assessment and diagnosis will be noted and if risks have been identified, a crisis plan may need to be carried out urgently.

If the risks are low, then cases will be discussed in either the daily MDT huddle or the weekly formulation meetings. Chaired by either a nurse or a psychologist, the huddle (where cases are analysed and evaluated) is an attempt to determine appropriate treatment interventions, challenge possible misconceptions about the patient and where multiple professionals such as pharmacists, occupational therapists, social workers will offer their input. Membership to the huddle is high which guarantees robust discussion with a genuine motivation to take time in unpacking the patient's inner world.

A noted change since engaging elements of formulation within these clinical spaces has been a significant reduction in the number of first appointments booked with the psychiatrist as case formulation has made it noticeably easier to identify which biopsychosocial interventions may be the most beneficial.

If a service user has specifically requested a diagnostic assessment, then that's what will be offered to them. However, there is a keenness to move away from entrenched pathology which reinforces the idea that there is something "wrong" with the person or that the psychiatrist knows best. Instead, there may be a focus on social recovery or an intervention from the pharmacist or to enlist the help of a floating support service.

Another positive has been that referrals to other internal and external services are accepted far more quickly as due to case formulation, a referral can be made verbally instead of having to complete lengthy referral documents. Some specialist services no longer require a formalised diagnosis because they are a part of the discussion which helps to qualify what the formulation has led to.

The challenges that have arisen are that given the complexity of some of the cases, formulation can be time consuming, so not many cases can be discussed, and meetings can often run over time.

There may also be a clash of opinions sometimes as each professional may not share the same understanding of the service user's difficulties or agree with the action planning.

What has been key in addressing these challenges is having a good chairperson who has gone through the clinical information prior to the huddle, identified urgent risks and is then able to provide a clear sense of focus and direction.

To formally embed the framework of formulation into clinical practice, further training should be offered specifically to mental health nurses throughout their careers. This will increase their confidence in using the approach and support integrative, holistic working with our service users.

Jeanette Jones-Bragg—Band 8 Service Manager, Adult Community Mental Health

I see formulation as a collaborative process that promotes shared understanding with the patient (using the patient's narrative) and to ensure their care is meaningful. I use a model of formulation (5Ps) and this can help to navigate and understand the patient's immediate problems and longer-term challenges. I also use safety plans.

I do experience mental health nurses undertaking formulation, but it is not a common process undertaken by nurses as it is seen as a psychologist role.

The service user is involved throughout the process of formulation, from the explanation to the reviews and the formulation is agreed with the patient. It is best completed face to face.

I think training is essential and promotes nurses facilitating formulations. It needs to be seen as an important skill for nurses and for other professionals to understand this as a nursing skill.

Lynette Robinson—Band 8 Senior Clinical Lead, Planned Care

I am a senior clinical lead in planned care mental health (community) and also work within the mental health collaborative ICB (Integrated Care Board).

I consider my understanding of formulation is good but I haven't practised for a while. I received training on formulation via a previous trust and 1:1 with a psychologist. I have completed dual diagnosis training and received content on the academic principles of formulation.

I undertook formulation previously in another role. I am now involved via multidisciplinary team discussion. I do experience seeing mental health nurses undertaking formulation within Early Intervention in Psychosis Services.

From my experience, service users are involved in formulation via the interview stage and are then presented with the formulation. I would not consider this a collaborative process.

I think more training is required for nurses, as formulation tends to be seen as a psychological professions' role.

Emma Ballantyne—Mental Health and Wellbeing Practitioner (MHWP) Working in a Primary Care Mental Health Hub

Formulation helps the service user and clinician to understand what intervention is required and what is maintaining their current problem. It also helps gather information about what led to the problem. Formulation helps with understanding the link between our thoughts, feelings and behaviours and how emotions make themselves known to us by physical sensations within the body. Formulation also explains to the service user how changing an area of the 5 areas formulation can help break this cycle for example behaviour. It can be helpful in explaining vicious cycles and inspire people to recognise areas they can change.

As a MHWP we complete low intensity formulations including a 5Ps and 5 areas formulation. As part of our 5Ps formulation we also discuss risk and complete a brief safety plan if required. Risk is covered at each session and monitored throughout interventions and safety plans are reviewed accordingly.

Within our team, nurses do not complete formulations. Some nurses go on to complete further training in CBT where they will use formulations. Our nurses complete assessments based on the DIALOG assessment tool and complete brief interventions prior to service users being allocated to a psychological professional (either low intensity or high intensity based on need).

The service user is involved in the 5 areas formulation. The diagram is shown to them and explained so they understand the link between the areas. The 5Ps assessment is completed collaboratively with the service user. Language is changed to help with understanding, for example, how was your childhood growing up? (predisposing) Do you think there is anything which triggered your mental health to decline (precipitating) and what do you feel is keeping you stuck (perpetuating)? The service user also completes their own problem statement which helps lead into the 5 areas formulation. SMART goals are also completed collaboratively to help the service user improve areas of their life and help break their maintenance cycle.

I think it would be helpful for nurses and social workers (Mental Health Practitioners) within the team to have a better understanding of formulation to help with assessments.

Bridget Flynn—Highly Specialist Psychological Therapist, Adult Community Mental Health and Clinical Lecturer for the Mental Health and Wellbeing Practitioner (MHWP) Programme, Specialist Adult Mental Health

My role/title is Highly Specialist Psychological Therapist for three days of my working week. I work in an Adult Community Mental Health team in a large town. I am also a lecturer on the MHWP programme in Higher Education for the other two days of my working week.

In my first role in practice, a formulation involves the gathering of a complete set of information about the client's life to date. It can include physical, psychological and social history. We use the 5Ps template and this incorporates presenting problems, predisposing issues, precipitating issues, perpetuating issues and protective factors. Once all this information is gathered, we sit down with the client and their significant others (if the client wants them there) to plan what are our next steps and matching what we as a service can offer the client. In the second area of work the word "formulation" is used to describe the 5-aspects model from Cognitive Behaviour Therapy. This gathers information about a specific problem a client has and then with the collaboration of the client, is used to identify the service the clinician can offer the client to address their current needs.

I undertake formulations in different stages. In my role as psychological therapist, I lead formulation meetings with the clients, their lead professionals (LP)/care co-ordinator (CC) and any significant other they choose to attend the meeting. I join at the stage where the client and their LP/CC have created the document with the 5Ps. I will have reviewed the document before the meeting. We all sit down, go through the document and discuss what the client wants and what we are able to provide. We negotiate what our next steps are. In my role as psychological therapist I use the 5-areas model, and the interpersonal safety and risk assessments and summaries during most of my 1:1 sessions.

The mental health nurses do participate in the formulation process in my first role mentioned above. They are the LPs or the CCs. They are the ones, together with the clients, who prepare the formulation document prior to the formulation meeting. In the Adult Community Mental Health Team there is a 12-week "pathway" process. In that time the LP/CC will meet with the client on a number of occasions to collect the information required for the formulation. They will also use techniques such as reading through any previous notes we may have gathered on the client, arranging physical health assessments and getting GP summaries. All this information goes in to the formulation.

The service user is involved every step of the way, from being accepted by the team and being allocated a LP/CC. They are invited to the meetings mentioned above to gather all the information using the 5Ps and whatever other assessment that is indicated by their presentation for example risk assessments, safety planning and summary, 5-areas model, SMART goal setting, to mention but a few. The formulation document is the central assessment document for this process and the client is involved in its creation. Then when the formulation meeting happens, the client is present, and their views are actively sought out and encouraged. The negotiation about what is the next step is very much guided by what they have requested from the service. My second role as a clinical lecturer is not patient facing. The service users in this case are the students. They are learning how to do the assessments using the 5P, and 5-aspects models.

In the Adult Community Mental Health Team, we are lucky to have other disciplines involved. We have Social Workers, Nurse Associates and a MHWP. People who work in these roles function as LP as well as the Mental Health Nurses on the team. I do think training would be helpful for everyone involved. It is one of the areas that new staff need a lot of guidance on when they start with the team. I do believe that is because the process of formulation differs from team to team and from area to area, for example community and inpatient. New staff who were recently trained as nurses, social workers, or MHWPs talk about their experiences in other teams where formulations are done completely differently. We have developed the technique and process we use over a number of years. Who is to say that we are right? There is always room for improvement.

Natalie Turner—Clinical Associate Psychologist Working in Primary Care Mental Health

I am a Clinical Associate Psychologist working in Primary Care Mental Health. My understanding of formulation is that it is a more person-centred, holistic alternative to diagnosis. It allows people to gain an understanding of how their past experiences have influenced their current ways of thinking, feeling, and behaving, which may be maintaining current mental health difficulties.

I do undertake formulation. I complete the 5 areas formulation with patients presenting with a range of mental health difficulties including anxiety, depression and complex emotional needs. This helps them to understand how they respond to triggers in terms of their thoughts, feelings, and behaviours, and how this response may act to maintain a vicious cycle. I will use this formulation to explore potential skills and techniques that will help them cope in the longer term and interrupt the vicious cycle. I also complete longitudinal formulations with patients with difficult and traumatic early experiences. This helps us to understand how their negative core beliefs about themselves, the world, and others, may be contributing to their current difficulties.

We have mental health nurses in our MDT. They use formulation to understand what is maintaining difficulties at the present moment to help us decide the most appropriate treatment pathway, for example psychological intervention, housing support, social inclusion etc.

When completing a 5 areas or longitudinal formulation, I use Socratic questioning and the downward arrow technique within sessions to help patients identify their beliefs and vicious cycles. I encourage patients to take their formulations home, recognising and recording when they notice these patterns being played out in their day-to-day life. I emphasise that a formulation is adaptable and should be added to throughout the course of intervention and beyond. It is a therapy tool in itself to help recognise unhelpful patterns of thinking and behaving, and to try to replace this with more helpful thoughts and behaviours.

I believe patients understand their difficulties more with a formulation compared to a diagnosis, so I am happy to see this moment within mental health. However, not every professional/service is on the same page. I think more formulation training for more medical staff, for example psychiatrists, would benefit mental health services overall.

ANALYSIS AND SUMMARY OF KEY THEMES OF ACCOUNTS

The Mental Health Nursing Role and Formulation

As part of the six core values of nursing practice, "Care" is the first value on the list as there is an expectation that nurses *will put the patient at the heart of everything we do* (NHS England, 2016). For nurses to ensure that care is meaningful, care needs to be specific to service users' needs and demands that cross all areas of practice. High-quality standards of nursing care delivery are essential (Baillie, 2017).

Models of formulation such as the 5Ps (Macneil et al., 2012) take into account several contributing factors that consider the challenges faced by the service user and find ways in which to conceptualise them holistically. With this in mind, it could be suggested that formulation is already an established component in mental health nursing as we engage within an ongoing process of collaborative assessment with service users and offer evidence-based interventions. Whether consciously or not, individual formulation takes place almost systemically, as biopsychosocial assessments are carried out by a nurse whether in an A&E mental health liaison department, a home treatment/crisis team or sitting within a GP practice. These are likely to begin with looking at the "presenting problem".

Risk assessments or risk management plans delve into the precipitating and predisposing influences which may impact a person's ability to keep themselves safe. Plans will also identify which future factors may be protective or mitigating. This information gathering takes place throughout assessments and will go on to inform which evidence-based intervention will be offered.

Throughout this chapter, practitioners have discussed the advantages of using formulation either as part of a dynamic risk assessment individually or within a multidisciplinary team structure that facilitates spaces for robust discussions pertaining to complex cases. Baird et al. (2017) suggest that service users presenting with complex presentations such as those with comorbidities benefit from formulation as it can help to deepen the therapeutic alliance between patient and practitioner. However, researchers have argued that community-based multidisciplinary teams that utilise a formulation-based approach were only really successful when the role of formulation was clearly defined and, when there was a sharing of perspectives and knowledge across the different disciplines (Tinemakomboreroashe, 2015).

Some mental health teams have embedded formulation into their multidisciplinary core. Some of the practitioner accounts in this chapter have highlighted that psychologists do take the lead on formulation approaches with regard to facilitation and training and will share their knowledge and skills with the wider team. This may lead to a team becoming more "psychologically minded" which insinuates that the team is less "diagnostically" led and more open to considering the other important aspects of a service user's life such as cultural, psychosocial or occupational influences. This appears to be in contrast to McKenna et al. (2022) who argue that due to a lack of training and poor understanding of its meaning, formulation in community mental health settings are often dismissed.

What has created a shift within community mental health culture has been that over time, the MDT has helped to reposition the power balance away from the psychiatrist and disperse it amongst the other health care professionals that sit within the team (Orovwuje, 2008). Although MDTs are now very much standard practice, the NHS People Plan (2021) once again outlines an ambition to continue to address the breaking down of barriers within teams and across organisations to ensure that those with health conditions are able to access support. Part of that work has been to improve communication and deepen trust within the team, to have a diverse workforce and greater understanding around roles (NHS England, 2020).

It can be considered that when thinking about the mental health nurse role and multidisciplinary power dynamics, having a consultant psychiatrist who is not medical model-led and who is keen to have space to think, unpack and share skills interprofessionally, can greatly help the team to be less diagnostically entrenched. As nurses, we form an integral part of multidisciplinary working and engage within the ongoing process of the assessment of patients and offering of evidence-based interventions, but we perform a number of other duties too which adds complexity to an already very challenging role.

Mental health nurses have become "biopsychosocial interventionists" (Painter, 2021) because we have developed and accrued skills from other fields and disciplines. Some practitioners would say that our roles are more "fluid" and less to do with for example facilitating a depot clinic and more geared towards offering psychologically informed interventions with a trauma focused lens. For some, this may lead to concerns that formulation is something "extra" that nurses would need to learn or that formulation is viewed by some as a tick box exercise.

This chapter has suggested that some mental health nurses are already implicitly using formulation as part of their work but some may not be explicitly saying so, and this could be due to a number of reasons. Anecdotally and from experience, we may conclude that nurses are not given the same amount of time as other disciplines to think and reflect following what can often be an in-depth, possibly distressing assessment. We are expected to move onto *the next thing* or are rushing off to *fight crisis fires*. This may undermine confidence in our skills in the using of other approaches and tools such as formulation which may prompt us to seek out more formalised training.

Risk Assessment, Management and Formulation

There appears little doubt that as mental health nurses we strive to make sense and gain a wider understanding of our patients' distress, what drives this and fundamentally how we can intervene to support individual recovery, which formulation as a process can facilitate. Reflecting on the clinical views in this chapter, albeit different approaches and use of formulation exist, there appears to be a general "wanting to gain a deeper understanding" consensus coupled with some concerns around a lack of formulation training and time to complete this important work with clients.

Formulation is more than gathering information, it is a process of collaborative working with a client for a biopsychosocial understanding of their problem, what keeps the problem going, exploring what helps and what doesn't, whilst drawing on the impact of the client's thoughts, feelings and behaviours. Alongside the knowledge on diagnosis, mental health nurses' use of formulation provides clients with an individualised trauma informed intervention, where the mental health nurse elicits "what happened to you", rather than a sole focus on symptoms aligned to diagnostic medical criteria (Centre for Healthcare Strategies, 2021; Johnstone, 2018).

Risk assessment and risk management remains an essential component of a mental health nurses' holistic assessment and intervention with their client. The process of unstructured clinical judgement, actuarial methods and structured clinical judgement are used to conduct a risk assessment and indicate a risk management plan (Ahmed et al., 2021). The National Confidential Inquiry into suicide and safety in mental health (University of Manchester, 2021, updated 2024) outlines key messages in respect of; not relying on tools to predict risk, the importance of family and carer involvement and collaborative assessment with safety planning which is individual to a client and their presenting problem. Risk formulation can provide the framework for client involvement in gaining an understanding of the risks individual to them. If we consider the 5Ps model of formulation (Macneil et al., 2012), this provides the framework from which information can be elicited from a client about their risk, provide insight into historical factors and develop a shared understanding of the risk through open dialogue. We can see in this chapter, evidence that formulation is being used by mental health nurses in practice, with assessments structured around the essence of formulation, which facilitates means to support and understanding with their clients, in order to provide the most appropriate interventions (risk management plan) to minimise risk and improve outcomes. Consideration maybe needs to be taken into this way of introducing formulation in risk assessments and indeed mental health nursing practice.

Using a model of formulation to gather information collaboratively and then knowing what to do with that information in terms of attaching psychological theory could be two separate aspects of this process. As seen in the clinician contributions to this chapter, the need for education around the use and application of formulation could be considered essential if we want to see formulation embedded in routine contemporary mental health nursing practice.

The Multidisciplinary Team and Formulation

The Association of Clinical Psychologists (ACP UK, 2022) describes the purpose of team formulation as "supporting team members to develop a biopsychosocial, nonjudgmental understanding of service users' needs and difficulties, enabling compassionate care, and collaborative, strengths-based care planning". This is a positive of using team formulation identified in the accounts from practitioners. Practitioners pick out the importance of the service user being central to the formulation, understanding their story. When a person is unable/does not want to participate in team formulation processes (for various reasons—commonly risk of re-traumatisation), staff identify the need to have robust discussions around the person and understanding their "inner world". Recognising the need to share the information and decision making with the service user in an appropriate way is seen as essential (and where possible, or if appropriate with family members/advocates).

From the presented practitioner accounts in this chapter, it has been identified that there are variations on what "team formulation" looks like in different services. Some have formal systems and others more informal (huddle, team discussions, group discussions). Informal sharing of ideas is seen as important, especially in a "hectic" environment (Christofides et al., 2012). Though in contrast, Stratton and Tan (2019) found that following a structured framework in the form of cognitive analytic team (CAT) formulation was beneficial for self reflection and working with complex mental health problems.

Practitioner accounts reflecting on team formulation recognise the benefits when working with complex cases involving understanding and working with behaviours that challenge. Team formulation helps the team to discuss and analyse the experiences of the person and helps them to approach the care of the person in a trauma informed way. This has not always been the case in traditional mental health services. This can help to reduce some of the stigma around people that are "stuck in the system" that exists within services and help to re-evaluate care/support/intervention options. This is reflected in research showing positive results for the staff's understanding, their (staff) belief in being able to help "complex mental health", building more empathy, understanding service users' difficulties and feeling less stuck with challenging cases, resulting in better more focused plans of care (Bealey et al., 2021; Christofides et al., 2012; Stratton & Tan, 2019). Team formulation has shown that staff feel more validated and more confident in their care delivery and decisions (Bealey et al., 2021). They identify that shared decision making and sharing the emotional impact of working with complex mental health, "Seeing service users more as people, less as patients", improved compassion and helped staff feel more equal, rather than a hierarchical team and decreasing "blame culture" when everyone is involved.

There are also some variations as to who makes up the MDT in a team formulation depending on which service people are working in. Some research studies identified that having more roles involved helped to improve access to services (Bealey et al., 2021). This is because when they (other roles) have been involved in the formulation, they have an oversight of the "whole person" and are then more likely to accept the person into the right service/care/intervention for their need, without necessarily needing a diagnosis and further referrals. This is very beneficial to service users. Some services do use team formulation to inform the diagnostic process, if this is required. There is recognition (Bealey et al., 2021) that formulation can go alongside diagnosis—which is sometimes needed to inform the medication that might be needed and access to some services requires a diagnosis.

Though overall team formulation is seen as a positive approach to formulation there are some problems with it. Having different roles and viewpoints on a person's care can come with difference of opinions on care. There needs to be an understanding of different people's roles and responsibilities. Who makes up the "team" varies in different settings, depending on various reasons (such as the design, location, skill mix of the team) resulting in a postcode lottery of what type of services and approach to formulation a person receives. Some services are still embedded in more traditional modes and models of care (i.e. medical models), and this can be at odds with the ethos of formulation, reflected in a study by Stratton and Tan (2019).

There is also some debate about the lead role in facilitating the team formulation. Most of the research centres on psychologists facilitating team formulation, and it is viewed as their role (Stratton & Tan, 2019). This is not the case in practice and there needs to be more recognition and research into who is the most suitable person to facilitate. From practitioners' accounts, this varies in services. In some services, the staff member most involved with the service user facilitates, in other services it is still seen as a psychologist's role.

Other issues that have been identified have been staff not speaking up in sessions, so the more dominant voices or roles are the ones that are heard and therefore influence the outcomes more. Another consideration is staff feeling that they do not have enough knowledge of the service user, and so are afraid to speak up and the team dynamics (or politics as referred to in the practitioner accounts) prevent staff from contributing (Bealey et al., 2021; Christofides et al., 2012; Stratton & Tan, 2019).

Time and training are also identified as an issue. Not everyone is trained in formulation and does not understand the purpose of team formulation, or value it. Not all health trusts have given training to staff regarding team formulation and if staff do not understand it and recognise the benefits then it will not be prioritised or attended when services are overstretched.

The research into team formulation tends to be mostly from staff experience and service evaluations (Stratton & Tan, 2019). ACP UK (2022) call for further research into the impact of team formulation on the service user, and MDT attitudes of team formulation. This would further strengthen the evidence base for the need for team formulation within all mental health care services.

Personal Recovery Focused Approaches and Formulation

This chapter has captured views from mental health nurses incorporating other multidisciplinary practitioners involved in formulation. At the heart of many practitioner views expressed and within this subsequent themes discussion is the posing question *"...but who is the formulation for and why?"* We feel it important to consider this question in all forms of formulation to ascertain if the formulation stems from a collaboration between distressed person/person with presenting problem to be supported with exploration—to then move forward with aims of improving their situation. Alternatively, is the formulation a tool to support professionals in their problem solving and understanding of how to support an individual with their presenting problems? (The practitioner accounts in this chapter demonstrate reflections and practice in these areas.)

How do we then communicate how formulation may be utilised *to the client* as part of their care/support approach? Do we or do we not explain this to the client? Do we talk about these considerations with other professionals and in what forum? Such questions and processes around using formulation may need further thought and also in consideration of how formulation practice could be utilised more as central to supporting personal recovery approaches. Having these more direct conversations and discussions between service professionals and clients about what formulation can be and how it may support what people want in their lives, may lead to more collaborative communication and may help to redress power imbalances that we know historically have been underlying mental health service approaches and which still continue in differing guises.

Although personal recovery has been an underpinning premise to this book, it may be helpful to again reiterate that by personal recovery we are making reference to what is important to the individual and their personal growth and optimising daily living experiences. It has been described as; *"a way of living a satisfying, hopeful, and contributing life, even with any limitations caused by illness"* (Anthony, 1993, p. 17; Leamy et al., 2023, p. 2). Practitioner accounts have highlighted that formulation practice gives the opportunity to begin trying to gain an understanding of the individual and what may help them. This may sound like a logical aim and one that should have always been inherent in mental health care, but powerful accounts from those with lived experience bring home to us when this has not happened. Pat Deegan has talked about her experience of being told as a senior in high school that she had schizophrenia and that she would be sick for the rest of her life as well as needing to take high doses of antipsychotic medication for the rest of her life (Deegan, 2023). She was also told to avoid anything stressful (like school) and given the overall message that really all of her hopes and dreams were over and all she could do was exist from day to day. Pat calls this a *prognosis of doom* and passionately talks about the importance of hanging on to our hopes and dreams, referring to them as the stars that guide us in our recovery journeys. Many practitioner accounts in this chapter when talking about formulation have presented an outlook and focus on the importance of collaborating and joining the client on an exploration of their journey. We can only imagine what a pessimistic message and outlook such as that conveyed to Pat would have on ourselves either as someone experiencing a mental health problem or a practitioner who believed there was no hope for the future for someone we were supporting.

When considering using formulation approaches and how this can fully integrate into underpinning aims of supporting personal recovery in the person we are helping, we can deduce it is also important to think of our own recovery needs as practitioners. In the introductory chapter to this book, the editors (Vickie and Lolita) talked about their recognition that they often slipped back in to medical/psychiatric language whilst still attempting to retain a more trauma informed recognition of a client's presenting problems. They reflected on this and concluded this was because many areas they had held nursing positions within had been underpinned by a psychiatric diagnostic model (as well as practising within nursing/MDT led teams) and therefore this language was somewhat engrained and part of them. As has been highlighted in this book chapter, there is also a diversity of experiences in formulation practice and outlooks across the roles of mental health nurses which also link to underpinning dynamics in MDT practice and hierarchical or professional structures of how personal recovery outlooks now intertwine with mental health care provision. This can be identified as an important area for continued exploration. It may be helpful to consider further the *personal recovery of mental health professionals* to support them in being able to work within a personal recovery ethos (rather than a clinical recovery one, where reduction in symptoms and a focus on the diagnostic psychiatric model is often the focus) and to also be able to implement psychologically informed interventions and assessments, such as formulation.

There are already examples of how research and work is being undertaken in championing personal recovery by transforming mental health care (King's College London, 2023). Integral within these systems transformations are the integration of personal recovery frameworks such as CHIME (which stands for Connectedness, Hope, Identity, Meaning and purpose in life, Empowerment). This framework was identified by Leamy et al. (2011). The practitioner accounts in this chapter have highlighted well the often many hats mental health nurses are wearing, especially in roles such as care co-ordinators/lead professionals-practitioners, and how this can then lead to an experience of not having enough time and feeling overwhelmed. Practitioners have highlighted *training* as an important area for professional and role development in the area of formulation and there have been some, but not many accounts of the importance of *clinical supervision*. Both training and clinical supervision are areas which have been identified in the literature in supporting both psychologically informed practice and personal recovery approaches within mental health care. An example is a recent review which concluded that using a strengths-based approach is crucial in facilitating a safe space for service users by providing psychosocial interventions. Furthermore it was stated in this review that within inpatient units and community settings, there are still challenges in the understanding of recovery and how to provide recovery-orientated care (Chatwiriyaphong et al., 2024). NHS England, (2023, updated 2023) in their document, The Mental Health Nurses Handbook, state that supervision mechanisms must be in place for support and personal growth for mental health nurses, however in its section on Recovery Approaches and Transformation, it does not make any links or advise mental health nurses how supervision may support recovery orientated approaches. It would appear that rather than just mentioning contemporary approaches to improving mental health care within a mental health nurse's remit, further commitment and action is required to support mental health nurses in making this a reality and the provision of more in-depth guidance would be helpful.

INDICATIONS FOR FUTURE EXPLORATION, DEVELOPMENT AND RESEARCH

This chapter has undertaken a scoping exercise of mental health nurses' views and involvement in formulation, including the views of other practitioners and students involved in implementing formulation. From the accounts and themes identified, it is indicated a comprehensive piece of research would be helpful to involve a bigger representative sample of the practitioners who have offered their initial responses. It would also be helpful to identify more detailed case-study accounts of mental health nurses who have various forms of formulation fully integrated into their role and the services they work within. We would also like to identify the experiences of service users who have collaborated in formulation and what may have and not have been helpful to them in terms of working towards their recovery, whether this is considered clinical or personal. With many accounts in this chapter showing either an awareness and understanding of formulation and also involvement in formulation practice itself, it would appear this is an area for further development within mental health nursing practice with practitioners highlighting the importance of further training and support in developing their skills. We would also suggest that clinical supervision is another priority area in terms of formulation development and support for mental health nurses, although we acknowledge the challenges in accessing and engaging in clinical supervision in some areas of practice (Howard & Eddy-Imishue, 2020; Howard & Peirson, 2024; Masamha et al., 2022). In conclusion, we can state that using formulation is something that is not going away in terms of its use within mental health nursing roles. This is also supported by drivers such as the Advanced Practice Mental Health Curriculum and Capabilities Framework (Health Education England, 2022) which identifies formulation as an essential domain for mental health practitioners working at an advanced level.

> **Key Points for Reflection**
> This is a good opportunity to think about your own experiences and involvement in formulation. Please consider the following questions:
>
> 1. What are your own thoughts and experiences of using formulation?
> 2. Do you think the process of formulation is used by mental health nurses but is often not named "formulation?"
> 3. Have you observed or been involved in team formulation in your area of practice? What was your role in this? What members of the MDT were involved? Would any other team members' involvement have been beneficial?
> 4. What would be your own development needs for using formulation?

REFERENCES

Ahmed, N., Barlow, S., Reynold, L., Dret, N., Begum, F., Tuudah, E., & Simpson, A. (2021). *"Mental health professionals" perceived barriers and enablers to shared-decision making in risk assessment and risk management: A qualitative systematic review* (Vol. 21, p. 594). *BMC Psychiatry.*

Anthony, W. (1993). Recovery from mental illness: The guiding vision of the mental health service system in the 1990s. *Psychosocial Rehabilitation Journal, 16*(4), 11–23.

Association of Clinical Psychologists (ACP UK). (2022). *Team formulation: Key considerations in mental health services version 1.* ACP. acpuk.org.uk

Baillie, L. (2017). An exploration of the 6Cs as a set of values for nursing practice. *The British Journal of Nursing, 26*(10), 558–563. https://doi.org/10.12968/bjon.2017.26.10.558

Baird, J., Hyslop, A., Macfie, M., Stocks, R., & Van der Kleij, T. (2017). Clinical formulation: Where it came from, what it is and why it matters. *BJPsychAdvances, 23*(2), 95–103.

Bealey, R., Bowden, G., & Fisher, P. (2021). A systematic review of team formulations in multidisciplinary teams: Staff views and opinions. *Journal of Humanistic Psychology, 0*(0). https://doi.org/10.1177/00221678211043002

Boyle, G. (2008). The Mental Capacity Act 2005: Promoting the citizenship of people with dementia? *Social Care in the Community, 16*(5), 529–537.

British Psychological Society's Dementia Advisory Group. (2018). Evidence briefing: 'Behaviour that challenges' in dementia. *The British Psychological Society*, 1–4.

Centre for Healthcare Strategies. (2021). Retrieved March 7, 2024, from www.traumainformedcare.chcs.org/what-is-trauma-informed-care. (2021). *What is Trauma*

Informed care? Retrieved from Centre for Healthcare Strategies: www.traumain-formedcare.chcs.org/what-is-trauma-informed-care

Chatwiriyaphong, R., Moxham, L., Bosworth, R., & Kinghorn, G. (2024). The experience of healthcare professionals implementing recovery-oriented practice in mental health inpatient units: A qualitative evidence synthesis. *Journal of Psychiatric and Mental Health Nursing, 31*(3), 287–302. https://doi.org/10.1111/jpm.12985

Christofides, S., Johnstone, L., & Musa, M. (2012). 'Chipping in': Clinical psychologists' descriptions of their use of formulation in multidisciplinary team working. *Psychology and Psychotherapy, 85*(4), 424–435.

Cox, L. A. (2020). Use of individual formulation in mental health practice. *Mental Health Practice, 24.* https://doi.org/10.7748/mhp.2020.e1515

Deane, W., & Fain, J. (2015). Incorporating Peplau's theory of interpersonal relations to promote holistic communication between older adults and nursing students. *Journal of Holistic Nursing, 34*(1), 35–41.

Deegan, P. (2023, July 10). *Living our life, not our diagnosis.* YouTube: https://www.youtube.com/watch?v=A9trf_2KgwU

Geach, N., Moghaddam, N. G., & De Boos, D. (2017). A systematic review of team formulation in clinical psychology practice: Definition, implementation, and outcomes. *Psychology and Psychotherapy: Theory, Research and Practice, 91*(2), 186–215.

GOV UK. (2022). *Prime Minister's challenge on dementia 2020.* https://www.gov.uk/government/publications/prime-ministers-challenge-

Hartley, S. (2021). Using team formulation in mental health practice. *Mental Health Practice, 24*(2), 34–41.

Health Education England. (2022). *Advanced Practice Mental Health Curriculum and Capabilities Framework.* NHS HEE.

Holle, D., Halek, M., Holle, B., & Pinkert, C. (2017). Individualized formulation-led interventions for analyzing and managing challenging behavior of people with dementia – An integrative review. *Aging & Mental Health, 21*(12), 1229–1247.

Howard, V., & Eddy-Imishue, G. (2020). Factors influencing adequate and effective clinical supervision for inpatient mental health nurses' personal and professional development: An integrative review. *Journal of Psychiatric and Mental Health Nursing, 27*(5), 640–656. https://doi.org/10.1111/jpm.12604

Howard, V., & Peirson, J. (2024). Online group supervision as pedagogy: A qualitative inquiry of student mental health nurses' discourses and participation. *Issues in Mental Health Nursing.* https://doi.org/10.1080/01612840.2023.2283507

James, I. A., & Reichelt, K. (2019). Understanding people's needs: The 8-needs framework for the treatment of behaviours that challenge. Psychology of Older People. *The FPOP Bulletin, 147,* 24–30.

Johnstone, L. (2018). Psychological formulation as an alternative to psychiatric diagnosis. *Journal of Humanistic Psychology, 58*(1), 30–46.

Johnstone, L., & Dallos, R. (2006). *Formulation in psychology and psychotherapy: Making sense of people's problems.* Routledge.

Kaufmann, E., & Engel, S. (2014). Dementia and well-being: A conceptual framework based on Tom Kitwood's model of needs. *Dementia, 15*(4), 774–788.

King's College London. (2023, August 10). *Transforming mental health care by championing personal recovery.* Retrieved from King's College, London: https://www.kcl.ac.uk/news/spotlight/research-transforming-mental-health-care

Leamy, M., Bird, V., Le Boutillier, C., Williams, J., & Slade, M. (2011). Conceptual framework for personal recovery in mental health: systematic review and narrative synthesis. *British Journal of Psychiatry, 199*(6), 445–452. https://doi.org/10.1192/bjp.bp.110.083733

Leamy, M., Foye, U., Hirrich, A., Bjørgen, D., Silver, J., Simpson, A., et al. (2023). A systematic review of measures of the personal recovery orientation of mental health services and staff. *International Journal of Mental Health Systems, 17*(33). https://doi.org/10.1186/s13033-023-00600-y

Livingston, G. H.-M., Cooper, C., Costafreda, S., Dias, A., Fox, N. G., Howard, R., ... Orgeta, V. (2022). *Dementia prevention, intervention, and care: 2020 report of the Lancet Commission.*

Lloyd, M. (2010). *A practical guide to care planning in health and social care.* Open University Press.

Macneil, C., Hasty, M., Conus, P., & Berk, M. (2012). Is diagnosis enough to guide interventions in mental health? Using case formulation in clinical practice. *BMC Psychiatry, 10*(111). https://doi.org/10.1186/1741-7015-10-111

Masamha, R., Alfred, L., Harris, R., Bassett, S., Burden, S., & Gilmore, A. (2022). 'Barriers to overcoming the barriers': A scoping review exploring 30 years of clinical supervision literature. *Journal of Advanced Nursing, 78*(9), 2678–2692. https://doi.org/10.1111/jan.15283

McKenna, M., Brown, L., & Berry, K. (2022). Formulation-led care in care homes: Staff perspectives on this psychological approach to managing behaviour in dementia care. *International Journal of Older People Nursing, 17*(5).

McKenzie, E., & Brown, P. (2020). "Just see the person who is still a person (...) they still have feelings": Qualitative description of the skills required to establish therapeutic alliance with patients with a diagnosis of dementia. *International Journal of Mental Health Nursing, 30*(1), 274–285.

NCCMH. (2021). *The community mental health framework for adults and older adults.* NHS England.

NHS England. (2016). *Introducing the 6Cs.* NHS England.

NHS England. (2017). *The NHS long term plan.* NHS England.

NHS England. (2020). *WE ARE THE NHS: People Plan 2020/21 – Action for us all.* NHS England. www.england.nhs.uk/ournhspeople

NHS England. (2023). *The mental health nurse's handbook.* NHS England.

NICE. (2018). *Dementia: Assessment, management and support for people living with dementia and their carers. Guidance/ng97.*

NMC. (2018). The code: Professional standards of practice and behaviour for nurses and midwives.

Nyström, M. (2007). A patient-oriented perspective in existential issues: A theoretical argument for applying Peplau's interpersonal relation model in healthcare science and practice. *Scandinavian Journal of Caring Sciences, 21*(2), 282–288.

Orovwuje, P. (2008). Contemporary challenges in forensic mental health: The ingenuity of the multidisciplinary team. *Mental Health Review Journal, 13*(2), 24–34. https://doi.org/10.1108/13619322200800011

Painter, J. (2021, October 5). *'As mental health nurses, we are biopsychosocial specialists'.* Retrieved March 15, 2024, from Nursing Times: https://www.nursingtimes.net/opinion/as-mental-health-nurses-we-are-biopsychosocial-specialists-05-10-2021/

Spector, A., Orrell, M., Lattimer, M., Hoe, J., King, M., Harwood, K. Q., & Charlesworth, G. (2012). Cognitive behavioural therapy (CBT) for anxiety in people with dementia: Study protocol for a randomised controlled trial. *Trials, 13*(1).

Stott, J. (2018). *Cognitive behavioural therapy (CBT) for dementia.* Retrieved February 24, 2024, from Alzheimer's Society: https://www.alzheimers.org.uk/Care-and-cure-magazine/summer-18/cognitive-behavioural-therapy-cbt-dementia

Stratton, R., & Tan, R. (2019). *Cognitive analytic team formulation: Learning and challenges for multidisciplinary inpatient staff., 24*(2), 85–97. https://doi.org/10.1108/MHRJ-01-2019-0001

Surrey Place. (2024, February 25). *Behaviors That Challenge (BTC).* Retrieved from Developmental Disabilities Primary Care Program: https://ddprimarycare.surreyplace.ca/guidelines/mental-health/behaviours-that-challenge/

The University of Manchester. (2021). *The National Confidential Enquiry into suicide and safety in mental health (2021).* https://sites.manchester.ac.uk/ncish/

Tinemakomboreroashe, A. (2015). *Community mental health team members' perceptions of team formulation in practice.* Thesis, University of London. http://eprints.lincoln.ac.uk/id/eprint/22338/1/22338%20RPV1415%20Final%20with%20poster%20Tine%20Blee.pdf

Wang, L., Yang, L., Yu, L., Song, M., Zhao, X., Gao, Y., et al. (2016). Childhood physical neglect promotes development of mild cognitive impairment in old age: A case-control study. *Psychiatry Research, 242*, 13–18.

CHAPTER 9

Postscript

Vickie Howard and Lolita Alfred

INTRODUCTION

Each chapter of this book has highlighted different perspectives of what the human experience of distress might look like. It has also gone some way towards exploring equally varied means of understanding individual distress and leaning on formulation as the lynch pin between assessment and interventions. What this book has also shown is the importance of considering always, how we can enhance practice in a mental health nursing context, but also in a team context where mental health nurses, other professionals, the individuals experiencing struggles with their mental health and their family/carers can work together and interconnect.

This final chapter of the book incorporates key themes from the previous chapters. We hope this may spark your thoughts and further curiosity for your practice and/or experiences of what you will take away from this book. We are also offering some critical viewpoints here, again for your own consideration and to reflect on whether these are issues or concerns for you or alternatively you disagree with these and have alternative outlooks.

V. Howard (✉)
Faculty of Health Sciences, University of Hull, Hull, UK
e-mail: V.Howard@Hull.ac.uk

L. Alfred
School of Health and Psychological Sciences, City, University of London, London, UK
e-mail: Lolita.Alfred@city.ac.uk

A SUMMARY OF KEY THEMES ON FORMULATION FROM THE PREVIOUS CHAPTERS—STANDING BACK, CONSIDERING AND LEARNING

What We Have Learnt as the Book Editors

As book editors who are nurses and nurse educators—engaging in reflection is a key part of our practice, and a requirement for revalidation to maintain the currency of our registration with the Nursing and Midwifery Council. This postscript provides an account of our reflections on the several meaningful and important points for us during and at the culmination of this book. Firstly, we would like to highlight the energies and personal investments that all involved in the writing and production of each chapter have engaged in. We and the chapter authors were not aware of many of the challenges we would face in putting our thoughts and experiences down on paper in the way in which we have. Amongst ourselves we have had discussions about how the writing of each chapter has brought about our own realisations on areas of discomfort, uncertainty and unexpected questions we needed to ask ourselves. Sometimes we have had to tread carefully and give time, recognising that our own wellbeing comes first. Our collaborations have sometimes required breaks to reflect, to take the next step in our writing journeys. This has often included reflections on ethical approaches and associated issues which have surfaced, for example considerations on navigating issues of confidentiality, anonymity and privacy. This book does not use a traditional textbook format and we have considered and learnt as we have gone along. Rather than third person detached content, it incorporates many first person personal, autobiographical accounts and as such these accounts have been re-visited with contributors to check they are still happy for them to be used. Similarly, considered processes for discussion with the formulation content have been re-visited, and revised. In a way, this represents that the subject of our explorations—Formulation—can and does change over time, because human beings have different experiences which evolve over time, and as we learn about ourselves; what contributes to struggles with mental health and what enhances emotional wellbeing can also change over time. To help us with compassionate and considerate approaches, as identified in the introduction chapter, we have borrowed from 'autoethnography' as a means of writing about experiences and applying these to wider cultural, political and worldly influences. Although this book does not claim to be a work of autoethnographies, many of the chapters do cross over in this way of writing and learning and have greatly supported us in addressing ethical considerations. An example of this has been the consideration of 'relational ethics' (Couser, 2004; Ellis, 2007) throughout the writings in this book. By this we mean we have been considerate of how our writings may impact on others and our relationships with others and we have constantly reviewed this and sometimes made amendments to accounts if and when this has become apparent and '*the right thing to do*'.

Formulation, Concepts of Recovery and the Challenges Posed

We hope that each chapter presented in this book has given you food for thought about what 'recovery' means in differing contexts and to different people. We consider that the book has highlighted that formulation (no matter which theory it is underpinned by) can facilitate someone to tell their story about what has happened to them, what their current problem(s) are, the positive factors in their lives and considerations for moving forward. It can greatly contribute to the aim of *living well* amidst challenges or experiences which may persist.

Cixous (1993, p. 156) states: '*But there is no "conclusion" to be found in writing*'. We extend this notion to life too and see the good and bad as *the living human experience*. In addition, we can add that how mental health support is given or offered by health and social care services is constantly under both review and scrutiny. Currently, there is no definitive answer to how we can improve this with a magical end result in sight—only incremental steps forward can be ascertained as outlooks and beliefs about what mental health and associated support entails. We have attempted to demonstrate throughout this book how formulation practice and its underlying aims and values can be quite a big incremental step and how this may be more fully embraced in mental health nursing, leading to a more person-centred and/or family-centred approach in listening and responding to the people we are committed to supporting in their journeys.

Formulation, Safety and Beyond

Who is the formulation for? This is a question which has either overtly been discussed in this book or which may have sprung into the forefront of your own thinking as you have read through the chapters yourself. In particular *team formulation* has been discussed both in the research and literature (Chap. 2) and in the practitioner accounts of using formulation in Chap. 8. Sometimes this has been in the context of practitioner discussion either with or without *client* involvement. This has understandably been within the circumstances of a safe forum for practitioners to try to understand and make sense of an individual's difficulties. In some situations, it has been focused on concerns about the person and possible risks and safety issues. Some practitioners (Chap. 8) have identified formulation in the form of a 5Ps formulation that would be included in a safety plan. This, however, would include discussion with the *client*. To us, these are areas which would benefit from further research with regard to the benefits and any detrimental outcomes within the context of power (im)balance and both risk averse and positive risk-taking culture.

How Does All This Fit into the Progression of Mental Health Nursing

The developing multidisciplinary mental health workforce now more than ever places a spotlight on the specific roles and responsibilities of differing professional groups. Clinical psychology and psychological interventions/psychologically informed interventions have expanded to include other roles including associate and assistant psychologists, psychological wellbeing practitioners, education mental health practitioners and mental health and wellbeing practitioners. As well as registered mental health nurses, other roles connected to nursing include nursing associates, apprenticeship nurses (as student nurses) and assistant practitioners. The identification of new roles under professional disciplines is guided by development agendas, underpinned by the aims of improving the support and therapeutic interventions available to people experiencing emotional distress. In consideration of the mental health nursing role, longstanding assumptions and also ambiguities on what a mental health nurse 'does' appear to us as even more crucial in needing not only review but also essential exploration in how a mental health nurse gains support in developing their therapeutic skills. Key questions are: What is the reality with professional and personal development opportunities and routes for mental health nurses? What are national agendas here? The emphasis on career progression in reality appears to be through managerial responsibility rather than therapeutic expertise and the associated development of advanced skills. This may possibly link to the de-emphasis on leadership expertise when such roles as *clinical nurse specialist* and *nurse consultant* were valued and prominent in mental health nursing as a means of practice leadership through research. Consequently, such roles involved evidenced leadership roles in the facilitation and commitment to clinical supervision systems and supported mental health nursing involvement in practice development and research leadership. Senior nursing roles such as *modern matron* and *junior/associate matron* introduced increased monitoring in areas such as infection control and environmental standards in inpatient environments with some registered mental health nurses in these roles experiencing being removed from involvement connected to mental health priority areas or clinical mental healthcare, even though they had senior expertise in mental health nursing practice. It is important to pause and consider what these changes in senior nursing roles may mean for the perception of the mental health nursing role and the skills and purpose of such nursing roles.

Bringing the conversation back to formulation and the consideration of current and developing mental health nursing roles, we can reflect on why some mental health nurses do and do not experience this as part of their practice. Where a service builds in formulation as central to practice, for example using the 5Ps formulation model within the safety planning documentation or developing roles in psychosocial interventions (PSI), it is more likely to be utilised and by mental health nurses because it is a requisite. However, we can question whether using a formulation within a safety plan is viewed as a therapeutic tool for relationship building and therapeutic practice or a documentation 'must do' tick box exercise.

EMBRACING DIVERSITY

Diversity is a theme that threads through the chapters. This includes diversity of stories and experiences on the various forms of emotional distress; diversity of the individuals at the centre of the chapters, diversity of perspectives, formulation approaches, ways to help, theories to draw on, and diversity of the professionals involved. In Chaps. 1 and 6, there is the exploration of the PTMF, and how this embraces cultural diversity and diversity of experiences and expressions of distress. Boyle and Johnstone (2020) highlight that if emotional distress and behaviour are viewed as socially meaningful responses to adversity (as opposed to mental illness), then our responses will inevitably vary. They also add that there will however also be cross-cultural similarities in some instances—because we share fundamental human characteristics such as seeking close relationships, feeling sad when we experience loss, or feeling scared of being physically harmed, or angry when we are insulted or offended. How we can accommodate these is an important question to ask regardless of the approach we take to supporting individuals experiencing distress. With the increasingly globalised settings we live and work in comes the opportunity to embrace and harness the power of diversity. However, in order to do so requires some cultural awareness and cultural competence. In mental health settings as an example, this will mean enhancing training and support for cultural competence, but also enhancing services and treatment options so that they are relevant and beneficial for all individuals who require them regardless of their cultural or religious background. It is promising (as mentioned in Chap. 6) to see the steady rise in a body of work that explores culturally adapted therapy and approaches to enhancing mental health services so that they cater for all those who may benefit from their support.

RESEARCH GAPS

Literature identifies areas that could benefit from further research to enhance the body of evidence on formulation. These areas include research on efficacy, process and function of formulation, development and implementation of guidelines, and skills analyses and formulation training programmes (Rainforth & Laurenson, 2014). What has been indicated in gathering the perspectives, examples, and accounts of formulation throughout this book is that there is a language requirement in policy and associated guidance regarding when the word 'formulation' is used and how it is used according to the specificity of the formulation approach being referred to. It is far too easy to use this word as a generic term. Throughout this book, including within the introductory Chaps.

(1 and 2) and in the practice example Chaps. (3 and 8) a diversity in how formulation may be used and applied to mental health nursing practice has been demonstrated. Future steps to strengthen these examples include the presentation of further research studies which demonstrate how these formulation approaches have been applied in mental health nursing practice and their associated outcomes, combined with lived experience accounts.

CONSIDERATIONS FOR MENTAL HEALTH NURSE EDUCATION

Reflecting on the historical outlooks on the developing mental health nurse role may support us in establishing ways forward in using formulation within practice: The Thorn Initiative (in the UK) beginning around 1992, developed at a time when policy was progressing to meet the needs of people with serious mental illness. The Thorn Initiative included diploma and later degree programmes with core modules consisting of case management, family interventions and psychological/psychosocial interventions (PSI) (O'Carroll et al., 2004). This programme then broadened out further to see degrees in PSI being offered, based on a stress vulnerability model of mental illness and were designed to equip community mental health nurses with therapeutic skills to support those with severe mental health problems and their families. PSI has been identified to comprise of stress management, self-coping skills, relapse prevention and psychoeducation, as well as incorporating psychological therapies such as cognitive behavioural therapy (CBT) and/or motivational interviewing (Mullen, 2009). A review of educational programmes on psychosocial interventions found that 94% of programmes included specific teaching on structured assessment, formulation and the collaborative development of problem lists and goals (Mairs & Arkle, 2007). Although this review did not comment on the practice of formulation specifically, it indicated that PSI was beneficial because of its potential to enhance outcomes for those with psychosis who use services and their carers. It also highlighted that some students of PSI could experience problems in integrating PSI within their routine practice, with an obstacle cited as the lack of recognition of the value of PSI from colleagues and managers (Fadden, 1997). The issue of the integration of PSI in to care co-ordination roles has continued and is highlighted in Chap. 8. Happell et al. (2002) also identified that mental health nurses reported that there was no time to engage in these activities. In addition, specifically relating to inpatient mental healthcare, it has been identified that a trend developed towards observing patients rather than meaningfully engaging and interacting with them (Mullen, 2009). With formulation fitting in to PSI models and psychological interventions within this time frame of the early 1990s to the late 2000s, when higher education also reflected undergraduate and postgraduate education supporting advancement of PSI skills acquisition, the question can be posed—has this continued or changed direction for mental health nurses' professional development and attainment of therapeutic skills which would incorporate formulation?

The publication of the Mental Health Nursing Competence and Career Framework (Health Education England, November 2020, p. 4) had the intention of providing mental health nurses with a '...*much needed guide to sustain post-registration, postgraduate education and continuing professional development*'. It also intended to support those who were thinking about a career in nursing to consider mental health nursing. However, this framework does not grab the bull by the horns by tackling the intersection of drivers in mental healthcare from a service perspective and personal recovery perspective and indicate navigations for mental health nurses through historically driven hierarchical practices concerning psychiatry. It does not explicitly identify the curricula involved in post-registration, postgraduate and continuing professional development. The language of psychological interventions and PSI is non-evident and considering many educational postgraduate programmes not so long ago were prioritised in these areas, this is questionable. Furthermore, although 'formulation' is identified as a capability in the Advanced Practice Mental Health Curriculum and Capabilities Framework (Health Education England, 2022a), the specific knowledge and skills required in what the specifics of the formulation practice entail is not identified. This document advises that advanced practitioners should be able to construct formulations of patients' problems. Formulation is referred to in this document along with generic statements as, 'psychological, biological and social formulation'. There appears a need for further detail here of what this will look like. A review including recommendations for the future provision and development of the profession of mental health nursing (Health Education England, 2022b) called for an enhancement of the therapeutic relationship, a valuing of experiential knowledge and a promotion of the core skills of all mental health nurses. Though this is a strong starting point in calling for a more evidence-based and identified status of what mental healthcare delivery within mental health nursing involves—the established range of skills required in mental health nursing is not evident with the review surmising in Recommendation 8 that mental health nursing must become a more attractive profession with clear development pathways and opportunities at all levels. This still leaves the profession of mental health nursing as an ill-defined profession according to this review, still in need of further work and clarification of how to develop in the absence of a clear pathway to senior roles such as nurse consultant/approved clinician roles. We additionally feel that the mental health nursing role with regard to integrating psychologically informed approaches and PSI, of which formulation is a component has in some instances either taken a step backwards or left the discussion of what mental health nurses should be undertaking in their roles to support the distressed individuals they care for. This leaves mental health nurses without training and a pathway for development in these areas. For example, the transition from the focus being on PSI within postgraduate provision has moved to advanced nurse practitioner (ANP) or advanced practitioner (AP) training packages but without a clear indication on what this should entail from a mental health nursing perspective using therapeutic and psychologically informed skills. These are key factors and raise the possible underlying root causes of difficulties in retaining and recruiting mental health nurses in the profession—many potential student mental health nurses are drawn to mental health nursing because they envisage sitting and talking with someone who may be in distress and then using their skills therapeutically to support the person which should involve incorporating psychologically informed approaches. We have heard practitioner accounts in Chap. 8 which convey the many hats mental health nurses are wearing and the difficulty in gaining the time to implement what was once considered fundamental therapeutic work. As Health Education England (2022b) point out, the mental health nursing workforce in the UK has significantly reduced in the last decade with numbers similar to those at the start of the 2010s. Though a fuller exploration of the underlying reasons for this is required, there is already anecdotal evidence such as those mentioned here with regard to the challenges of the mental health nursing role being involved in an increasing broader collection of responsibilities which detract from the original reasons why compassionate individuals joined the profession.

As already identified, the word 'formulation' is mentioned generically in the aforementioned policy documentation, however how the word is being used is not clearly outlined and defined and no descriptive examples of its use are given. This further leaves the mental health nurse with unclear direction in how they can specifically develop their practice in the area of formulation. Looking at this from a positive perspective however may enable education providers a degree of autonomy in establishing what will be helpful from a practitioner and service user perspective within ANP programme curricula. ANP programmes were originally developed from a physical health perspective, however due to the parity of esteem agenda (Mental Health Taskforce, 2016) in recognising equally the mental health support needs as well as physical health of people, focussed mental health ANP programmes are now being developed (Allabyrne et al., 2020). A further step required involves explicitly identifying what the curricula of these programmes entail regarding mental health education.

WHAT THE FUTURE MAY HOLD

In conclusion, this book has been inspired by the many students we have worked with who were trying to grasp the theory we were teaching, while making sense of how different formulation practice happened in clinical areas. It is also inspired by the identification of a gap in research and education about formulation within a mental health nursing context, and the recognition of the need to strengthen the psychologically informed role that mental health nurses can facilitate in supporting individuals who may be experiencing emotional and psychological distress. We hope that this book will provide a concise, easy-to-understand reference point for the use of formulation in a mental health nursing context. Furthermore, we also hope the book will build momentum to develop the use of formulation further in mental health nursing practice and multidisciplinary teams—with the ultimate goal of understanding individual distress and supporting those we strive to help.

REFERENCES

Allabyrne, C., Chaplin, E., & Hardy, S. (2020). Advanced nursing practice in mental health: towards parity of esteem. *Nursing Times [Online], 116*, 21–23.

Boyle, M., & Johnstone, L. (2020). *The power threat meaning framework*. PCCS.

Cixous, H. (1993). *Three steps on the ladder of writing*. Columbia.

Couser, G. T. (2004). *Vulnerable subjects: Ethics and life writing*. Cornell University Press.

Ellis, C. (2007). Telling secrets, revealing lives: Relational ethics in research with intimate others. *Qualitative Inquiry, 13*(1), 3–29. https://doi.org/10.1177/1077800406294947

Fadden, G. (1997). Implementation of family interventions in routine clinical practice following staff training programs: A major cause for concern. *Journal of Mental Health, 6*(6), 599–612.

Happell, B., Manias, E., & Pinikahana, J. (2002). The role of the inpatient mental health nurse in facilitating patient adherence to medication regime. *International Journal of Mental Health Nursing, 11*, 251–259.

Health Education England. (2020). *Mental health nursing competence and career framework*. NHS Health Education England.

Health Education England. (2022a). *Advanced practice mental health curriculum and capabilities framework*. HEE.

Health Education England. (2022b). *Commitment and growth: Advancing mental health nursing now and for the future*. Health Education England.

Mairs, H., & Arkle, N. (2007). *Accredited training for psychosocial interventions for psychosis: A national survey*. NIMHE/CSIP National PSI Implementation Group.

Mental Health Taskforce. (2016). *The five year forward view for mental health*. NHS England.

Mullen, A. (2009). Mental health nurses establishing psychosocial interventions within acute inpatient settings. *International Journal of Mental Health Nursing, 18*(2), 83–90. https://doi.org/10.1111/j.1447-0349.2008.00578.x

O'Carroll, M., Raynor, L., & Young, N. (2004). Education and training in psychosocial interventions: A survey of Thorn Initiative course leaders. *Journal of Psychiatric and Mental Health Nursing*, 603–607.

Rainforth, M., & Laurenson, M. (2014). A literature review of case formulation to inform mental health practice. *Journal of Psychiatric & Mental Health Nursing, 21*(3), 206–213. https://doi.org/10.1111/jpm.12069

INDEX

© The Author(s), under exclusive license to Springer Nature Switzerland AG 2024
V. Howard, L. Alfred (eds.), *Formulation in Mental Health Nursing*, https://doi.org/10.1007/978-3-031-59956-9

Printed by Printforce, the Netherlands